Obesity:
THE MODERN FAMINE

*Discover the Underlying
Drivers of Weight and
Navigate Your Way to Health*

Obesity:
THE MODERN FAMINE

Dr. Kathy M. Campbell

**Based on DrKathy's popular
TEDx Talk**

Copyright © 2024 Kathy Campbell

All rights reserved. No part of this publication may be reproduced or transmitted in any form or by any means, electronic or mechanical, including photocopying, recording or any information storage or retrieval system, without prior permission in writing from the publishers.

This is a work of nonfiction. However, the names and identifying characteristics of certain individuals have been changed to protect their privacy, and dialogue has been reconstructed to the best of the author's recollection. The author and publisher of this book have used their best efforts in preparing the content and makes no representations or warranties with respect to the application or completeness of the content. The information is strictly for educational purposes. If one wishes to apply ideas contained within, the reader takes full responsibility for their actions.

This book is not intended to provide medical or pharmaceutical advice to individual readers. Dr. Kathy Campbell is a Doctor of Pharmacy (PharmD) who in no way represents herself as or replaces the advice of a Medical Doctor (MD) or a Doctor of Osteopathy (DO). To obtain medical advice the reader should consult a qualified and diverse team of medical and health professionals who will dispense specialized advice based upon each reader's medical history, current medical condition, and long-term health goals.

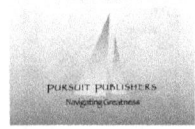

www.pursuitpublishers.com

ISBN: 979-8-9886274-0-1 (paperback)
ISBN: 979-8-9886274-1-8 (ebook)
ISBN: 979-8-9886274-2-5 (hardcover)
ISBN: 979-8-9886274-3-2 (audiobook)

Library of Congress Control Number: 2023919617

Printed in Tulsa, Oklahoma

Ordering Information:
Special discounts are available on quantity purchases by corporations, associations, and others. For details, contact www.pursuitpublishers.com

Names:	Campbell, Kathy M., author.
Title:	Obesity: the modern famine : discover the underlying drivers of weight and navigate your way to health / Dr. Kathy M. Campbell.
Description:	Tulsa, Oklahoma : Pursuit Publishers, [2024]	"Based on DrKathy's popular TEDx talk."	Includes bibliographical references.
Identifiers:	ISBN: 979-8-9886274-0-1 (paperback)	979-8-9886274-2-5 (hardcover)	979-8-9886274-1-8 (ebook)	979-8-9886274-3-2 (audiobook)	LCCN: 2023919617
Subjects:	LCSH: Obesity.	Self-care, Health.	Body weight.	Malnutrition.	Metabolism--Disorders.	Nutrition disorders.	Weight loss.	Reducing diets.	Obesity--Prevention.	Physical fitness--Nutritional aspects.	BISAC: HEALTH & FITNESS / General.	HEALTH & FITNESS / Diet & Nutrition / Weight Loss.	HEALTH & FITNESS / Healthy Living & Personal Hygiene.	HEALTH & FITNESS / Longevity.	HEALTH & FITNESS / Diseases & Conditions / General.
Classification:	LCC: RA645.O23 C36 2024	DDC: 362.1963/98--dc23

*This book is dedicated to the health of our children's children.
May we boldly and intentionally create a culture that produces health.*

TABLE OF CONTENTS

Introduction: Obesity as a Symptom of Our Modern World 1
Chapter 1: Obesity Is Our Modern Famine 7
Chapter 2: Famine of Knowledge. 9
Chapter 3: Famine of Nutrients 15
Chapter 4: Famine of Energy 23
Chapter 5: Famine of the Gut 29
Chapter 6: Famine of Stomach Acid 35
Chapter 7: Famine of Chemistry 47
Chapter 8: Famine of the Cell 61
Chapter 9: Famine of Fasting 67
Chapter 10: Famine of Flavor 79
Chapter 11: Famine of Fiber 83
Chapter 12: Famine of Water 89
Chapter 13: Famine of Oxygen 101
Chapter 14: Famine of Movement 107
Chapter 15: Famine of Heat and Cold 117
Chapter 16: Famine of Sunlight 121
Chapter 17: Famine of Darkness 131
Chapter 18: Famine of Sleep 135
Chapter 19: Famine of Connection 139
Chapter 20: Famine of Safety 145
Chapter 21: Famine of Support 151

Chapter 22: Famine of Relationships 155
Chapter 23: Famine of Hope 157
Chapter 24: Famine of Touch/Love 163
Chapter 25: Famine of Purpose 169
Chapter 26: NOURxISH! 175
Acknowledgements. 179
Endnotes 183

INTRODUCTION:
Obesity as a Symptom of Our Modern World

It is way too difficult to be healthy.

Calories are everywhere—and yet, we are constantly hungry. We live in a culture that reliably produces disease, as well as obesity, but blames the individual while simultaneously making it almost impossible to be any other way.

It is not your fault!

I want you to think of weight, obesity, not as a failing or weakness, but as a symptom of our body's function. This book will help you find clues to understanding your body's unique messages. What is your body trying to tell you?

It's the question I've been spending my life trying to answer, both as a pharmacist and someone who has lived with obesity.

My ultimate goal is to educate and empower you to craft a new culture, a new environment if you will, that produces the health required to live the life you want.

Contrast that intention with a typical trip to the doctor's office. You check in at the front desk, and after a wait, you get called back by the nurse. He checks your blood pressure, temperature, and then…your weight. **UGH!!** You came in because you feel tired and achy, and no matter what you try, you are having trouble losing weight. You've tried low-calorie diets. You tried keto. You tried doing extra exercise. But the weight did not budge—or worse, you gained weight despite all your efforts.

The doctor finally comes in. She sits at a computer and types as you begin to talk about *the* reason for the appointment (no longer are many allowed to discuss everything that concerns you). She notes that your temperature was low and that your blood pressure was slightly elevated. Eight minutes later, she is gone. Before she leaves, you have been given prescriptions for a blood-pressure medicine and an antidepressant, as well as a lecture about eating less and exercising more. Underneath this encounter is judgment. An unsaid bias. Your doctor didn't *say* "you are a fat lazy slob who does not want to be healthy." But research says she probably thought it.[1] You didn't imagine that poor treatment. Physicians, the medical community, and society in general treat weight as a problem within your power to change.[2] And based on that faulty judgment, the fact that your weight remains unchanged is *their* proof that you are at fault. To the patient, this judgment creates perceived stress, implies avoidance of care, engenders mistrust, and declares poor adherence to therapy.[3] People who are overweight are being neglected and abused by our medical system.

What is worse, **you believe it**. Even in the face of all of your efforts, you believe you are failing. You believe that you should be able to "do better." You believe that if you just eat less and exercise more, everything will be solved. It is a good thing that the doctor gave you an antidepressant! You're going need it after that encounter.

Both you and the medical community are wrong. These underlying judgments and assumptions are inaccurate and unfair. Worse, they distract from a deeper, more impactful clinical understanding. Would a doctor judge your character based on an elevated temperature? Would they blame or shame you if you came in with an infection and a temperature of 101? If you suddenly found yourself three inches shorter, would it be your fault?

The answer is likely no. Weight, like temperature, blood pressure, or height, are vital measurements of our body's function. If the body is having to adjust—having to survive—such adjustments will be seen in temperature, blood pressure, and, yes, weight. Each needs to be viewed in the context of the body's underlying function and survival.

Like temperature and blood pressure, OBESITY IS A SYMPTOM. Throughout this book, we will address what obesity, as a symptom, points to—the truth underneath those unique messages the body is sending. In the chapters ahead, we will be looking at many of the conditions that are coming together to create obesity and how you can create new conditions to produce different results.

Famine of Health

> *"Health-a state of complete physical, mental and social well-being and not merely the absence of disease and infirmity."*
> ~World Health Organization, 1948[4]

What is health? As the World Health Organization defined 75 years ago, health is not just the absence of disease.[5] My observation is that when patients want health, they really want vitality. They want a life where they can participate in that which is important to them. They want to play with their grandchildren or travel the world. They want to volunteer in their community. In order to participate, we must be able to function. Vitality is dependent on participation. Participation is dependent on function, therefore…

HEALTH=FUNCTION

Function is defined as "to operate in a normal way." My experience is that people just want to function well. We humans rarely think about our function until it is gone. There are four areas to consider when evaluating function: physical function, behavioral function, cognitive function, and what I am particularly trained in, metabolic function.

Pharmaceutical therapies are designed to impact metabolic function.[6] Many of my medical peers often think that I am anti-pharmaceutical therapies. This is not the case. I know what they do, how to help you achieve the best outcomes with their use, and how to avoid many of their negative effects if needed. I am not against the appropriate use of modern pharmaceutical therapies. I am, though, COMPLETELY AGAINST YOUR *NEEDING* THESE THERAPIES!! As a pharmacist who has practiced for 30+ years and an expert on modern pharmaceutical therapies and their impact on the body, I am clear that health is NOT taking 15 medications a day, but much closer to not NEEDING 15 medications a day. Unfortunately, accessing our current health care system (and the dollars locked within the insurance system) requires a diagnosis indicating often severe dysfunction. Within our current Western medical complex is little proactive support or structure for delaying the onset or the progression of these dysfunctions.[7] The current business model of health care will not help you function well or avoid becoming sick. Both will be up to you and me.☺

Challenges and Adaptations

Fundamentally, the human body is designed to survive and reproduce. We humans are the result of hundreds of thousands of years of challenges and adaptations. We have survived. ***YOU HAVE SURVIVED!*** For most of mankind's existence, getting enough food and surviving the elements was a 24/7 concern. Acquiring enough needed chemistries—protein, minerals, vitamins, water—consumed primitive human's every waking moment.

Our rhythms, instincts, and cravings evolved to seek out and consume as much of these critical chemistries as possible. It was very advantageous that a body be adaptable and efficient when food was scarce.[8] It was critical to be able to take a very little bit of available food and transform it into large amount of energy. It was also very beneficial for your offspring if they too, needed little food to survive. Over the generations we have developed into an efficient machine capable of surviving on little. We are designed to survive the ancient famine.

Modern life has thrown a wrench into that finely adapted system. Our primitive machines still require these critical chemistries (nutrients) to function, but our modern culture completely fails to meet our primitive demands. Arguably worse, the "foods" marketed by our culture provide toxic chemistries. In the modern world of excess, we live in lack—lack of nutrition, lack of sunlight, lack of oxygen, lack of water, and lack of connection. Lack of the chemistries critical for human function. Obesity is the appropriate biochemical symptom of our modern existence.

Why has our modern world lead us to this point, and what can we do to change these conditions? Is it just that we eat too many calories? Is it that we are lazy and not working hard enough? The answer is unequivocally **NO**! I hope you will realize that *you* are not the problem. Obesity is not the problem. Quite the contrary. Consider that obesity is the symptom and possibly even the body's survival solution to living in our modern world.

As you work through this book, see yourself. See where each issue may be pushing on your body. The cause is often hidden from us. See where your culture is contributing to your health. See where even a tiny shift can make a profound difference. That difference is health.

What Do You Want?

With any journey, it is important to have a destination in mind. I often will describe this journey like sailing a boat. Rarely does one sail in a straight line. One must harness the winds in a way that goes in the direction we want and does not sink the boat.

Begin to ask yourself "What do I want?" It's a simple question, but it can be extremely difficult to answer. When we were children, we could answer quickly and with confidence. But we often forget how to want and how to dream. In this journey, what you want will be the destination. That's where we'll aim our boat.

Naming your "destination" or your objective will guide your health journey. Do you want to feel confident wearing that dress you love? Do you want to be able to complete a 5K someday? Maybe a marathon? Maybe you wish to live independently? Or living a life of no pain? Maybe you simply want to live a longer, healthier life.

You don't have to be a 30-something or younger to step on board. Born in 1967, now 57 years old, I am an older mom. I love my daughters Emma (22) and Abby (19) completely and want a long, intimate relationship with them and their future children. My daughter Abby loves me dearly, but she is completely embarrassed by me when I dance. (For the record, I can dance quite well!) My health goal is to completely embarrass Abby at her daughter's wedding by twerking in the middle of the dance floor! I'll probably be around 90 years old then. To pull this off, I'll need to have the physical function of muscle and balance to dance, and I will need the mental function to enjoy knowing I am embarrassing Abby! In all seriousness, I want a long and vital relationship with my children and grandchildren.

As funny a visual as that scenario may be, there is another ***much deeper, much more critical*** component of this goal. Beyond my own muscle, balance, and brain health, Abby and her future partner must have the functional health to create a healthy human offspring. What drives me to write this book and share with you is my desire to create and cultivate a culture that produces health for you, your (and my) children, and their children.

CHAPTER 1:
Obesity Is Our Modern Famine

> *"If you do not change direction, you may end up where you are heading."*
>
> ~Lao Tzu

It's not your imagination. You are hungry all of the time. But you just ate! How can it be that you are hungry? And despite society's message to you that you should not be hungry, or that if you had a bit more willpower, everything would be perfect, the hunger is loud.

How is it that at a time when calories are everywhere, we can be so hungry? Well, just like our ancient ancestors, we are starving—we are deprived of that which our bodies **need** to function. I have termed this source of profound lack of what we need to function the **Modern Famine**. It is because we are "starving" that obesity is epidemic. It doesn't look like the kind of hunger where we have nothing to put into our mouths. It is a different kind of hunger. The kind of hunger that occurs when we lack what we need.

We are a bag of chemistry with a dose of God. The human body is a complex chemical machine designed to survive. Imagine driving a car with only two spark plugs, or with water in the gas tank, or with tires that lack air. The results would be a machine that did not work well, or at all. Much like how thirst is the message for the human machine to seek water, hunger is the message that the body needs to seek nutrients that it may not have. Throughout this book we are going to look at what those deficiencies or needs may be.

There are five fundamental "chemistries" needed for the human body to function: **food, oxygen, sunlight, water, and connection**. While simple, any disruption within each category will have enormous impacts on our function. Fundamentally, today's humans lack the chemicals to run our machine. We are starving at the cellular level.[9]

Health Strategy

- Know where you are going.
- Have a clear health goal. Explore and declare what you want for your health.

Practice

- DREAM! Dream BIG! What level of health and life would you want for the most precious person in your life? If money, time, and technology were no issue, what would that destination look like? Write it down in your health journal.

CHAPTER 2:

Famine of Knowledge

"Knowledge has power. It controls access to opportunity and advancement."

~Peter Drucker

Despite the abundance of "food" available, we are a profoundly misnourished, if not malnourished, society. How can that be? It's clearly a 21st century enigma.

The answer to that question requires the knowledge of what it takes to "feed" the human chemical machine. The common denominators are:

1. **Acquire** "necessary and appropriate" nutrition (grow, hunt, shop, knowledge)
2. **Prepare** food for consumption (dress, chop, cook)
3. **Consume** and digest food into usable nutrients (chew, digest, absorb)
4. **Utilize** nutrients at the cellular level (generate energy, repair, reproduce, metabolic function)
5. **Excrete**/get rid of what is not needed or is toxic (poop, pee, sweat, breath)

For most of human existence, humans had little choice on what to eat. Humans ate that which did not run away ... plants (tubers, nuts, green leaves, fruits), bugs, eggs, fish, small game, and larger, more difficult to hunt game if you had help (friends or family). We ate based on the seasons, what was available, and what we could get with the least amount of energy expended. If there were 500 calories on the plate, it often took 505 calories to get it there. Rarely was there too much food, and it required constant energy and diligence to obtain. During parts of the year where food may be plentiful, like the late summer, we were programmed to eat as much as possible to store precious fats in order to survive the impending starvation winter. Plants made up a major part of these diets, providing tremendous variety and nutrients that our body would use.[10]

Those who failed to gather enough food to operate their or their child's machine did not survive and did not live to reproduce. An efficient metabolism (engine) became a great advantage. Those with "thrifty genes"[11] survived! We all have been handed down the genetics to survive. We ate what nature provided, and what nature provided was the chemistry our machines needed.

My Personal Story

I am a heavy human born to heavy humans. I weighed 100 pounds at five years old (in 1972), 200 pounds at 10 years old, and 275 pounds when I graduated high school. My grandfather weighed over 350 pounds during the Great Depression. Obesity was common in our family at that time when obesity was estimated at 10% of the population.[12] My grandparents, parents, sisters, cousins were always the 1:10 humans who were obese.

It was nothing abnormal in our family, but I was unique in my community. I remember my mother commenting that I never had a weight problem until I had an appendectomy when I was five years old. My elementary school years (1970s) were filled with memories of visiting Dr.

H to be weighed and given these little yellow capsules (phentermine, a commonly used amphetamine diet pill). I was one of the tallest in my class in sixth grade but pretty much stopped growing at that point. Puberty hit, complete with extra weight and hair on my face and what would now be described as polycystic ovary syndrome.

During my childhood, I suffered little of the psychological damage typical of those who are overweight or obese,[13] possibly because of it being a family trait. I saw my own weight as normal based on my family's genetics. Never do I remember being shamed or belittled for being overweight by those closest to me. Most importantly, I was loved and accepted by my family regardless of my weight. My internal conversation about myself, programmed by my environment as I grew, was not negative in important ways. I was successful socially and academically, which led me to college, where I began my study as a scientist, on the road to becoming a pharmacist.

During college, I was placed on medications that accidentally stabilized my hormones. That coincidence continued what was to be quite the personal study of obesity—20 years of low-fat diet plans, weight-loss surgery, infertility. Each medical theory learned, each patient interaction filtered through the lens of a personal focus, study, and sensitivity. At times I weighed less, and at times I weighed more. Contrary to what society would have us all to believe, never was it about my not trying hard enough, having little willpower, or eating too much.

It is hard to imagine that our current cultural diet, The Standard American Diet (SAD), could be any further from what our human biology actually needs. The shift began long ago.

Prior to World War II, women spent more than two hours a day preparing food for the family.[14] Then, Rosie went out to rivet and did not return to the kitchen. The family garden began to be replaced by time-saving TV dinners and processed foods. I had the opportunity to visit the food exhibit at the National Museum of American History in D.C. to see Julia Child's kitchen.[15] As wonderful as that experience was, what caught my eye, of all things, was a picture of a minivan. Why was a minivan—the Chrysler Caravan to be exact—in a food exhibit at the Smithsonian Museum? Introduced in late 1983, the minivan was one of the first vehicles specifically designed to eat in and represented a catastrophic shift in how Americans consumed food.[16]

The 1980s also brought us the opportunity for cheap, fast food at every meal. What humans defined as food began to be determined by Wall Street and marketing companies, not by nature. No longer did our human nutrition consist of plant or protein, or even that classic recommendation of "vegetable, starch, and protein." We were light years away from our hunter-gatherer roots. The drive-thru era brought "kid's meals," the (un)foundational food of "nuggets, soda, and fries." It is no coincidence that menus of the most popular restaurants of today reflect the adult-size portions of kid's meals. This progression represents a catastrophic shift in what humans know as food.

During this time, our fundamental, ancestral knowledge of food began to disappear. Children no longer learned about food by working in the garden or on the family farm, or as they watched Grandma work her magic in the kitchen, or even in a high school home economics class. Instead, they learned about food from cereal advertisements during Saturday morning cartoons. The effort and the skill needed to prepare food began to be simplified or even eliminated by modern convenience and prepared food.

At about the same time, chaos erupted in the science of nutrition and medicine. During the 1960s, a debate arose in medicine as to the cause of heart disease. Compelling research pointed to the cardiovascular damage caused by sugar. Other research pointed to fat as being the driver of heart disease. Which one is it? Could it be both?

Unbeknownst to the public, strategic suppression of the research that sugar contributes to heart disease was perpetrated by the sugar industry. Harvard researchers were paid not to publish these studies. "Together with other recent analyses of sugar industry documents, our findings suggest the industry sponsored a research program in the 1960s and 1970s that successfully cast doubt about the hazards of sucrose while promoting fat as the dietary culprit in CHD (Coronary Heart Disease)."[17] The narrative of what we should eat was cunningly crafted by those who profited off your consumption of sugar…not based on what is necessary for health.

According to the Cleveland Clinic, not only are both fat and sugar generally bad for you (especially the amount in our Standard American Diet), but specifically saturated fats, trans fats, and added sugars.[18]

Those years began what I call the "SnackWell Revolution." Lots of cheap, convenient, high-sugar, low-nutrient food-like substances giving us the ***illusion of nutrition.*** The scientific narrative was now crafted by the industries profiting off your consumption with little interest in your health or function. I shudder to think of the lives impacted by this action—the heart attacks, strokes, diabetes, dementia, depression—the suffering.[19,20]

It does not help that our primitive human brains are wired to seek out that precious and rare fuel source called sugar. What a mess!

Health Strategy

- Assess and understand your physical, behavioral, cognitive, and metabolic function.

Practice

- Begin to collect the pieces of your puzzle. Gather information about you and your family's health history.

Include in this laboratory, pictures, histories, etc.
- What do you know about your parents' health and weight? Your grandparents?
- Start at the very beginning (conception) and develop a history or "timeline" of your health and weight.
- What has your body endured, and how has it reacted? C-section? Divorce? Injury? Antibiotic use? College? Broken leg? Marriage? These events and their resolutions are clues to what and how our bodies have survived.

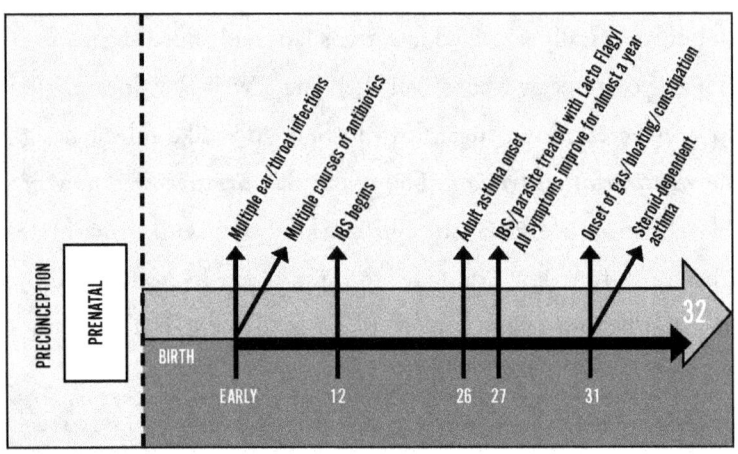

Health Timeline-drkathysays.com/timeline[21]

- Begin to assess the "chemistries" going into your body.
- Make a list of all medications, supplements, cosmetics, and foods that you routinely consume. It might help to look at receipts.

CHAPTER 3:
Famine of Nutrients

"Tell me what you eat and I will tell you what you are."
~Jean Anthelme Brillat-Savarin, 1825

What should we eat? It's a simple question, but the answer can get frustratingly complicated. We need enough of the appropriate chemistry to optimally run our machine. What *exactly* that consists of may actually be different for each of us.

The answer may depend on variables like genetics, health, family history, and environment. So, to get the right fuel for your body, you may need to study up on yourself. You are, after all, the only you and the expert of your bag of bones! Each of us is exquisitely unique! That being said, it's important to understand the basics of human function and nutrition.

Nutrients are substances that provide nourishment essential for growth and the maintenance of life. These compounds are essential to life and health, providing us with energy. They aid in the body's repair and growth and help to regulate chemical processes. An **essential nutrient** is one that the body needs that it can't create on its own. There are traditionally six essential nutrients split between two categories that the body needs to function properly.

Macro-nutrients (big nutrients)
- Carbohydrates (sugars)
- Lipids (fats)
- Protein[22,23]

Micro-nutrients (small nutrients)
- Vitamins
- Minerals
- Water

Plus the most essential nutrient often not considered...
- Oxygen[24]

Nutrients that can be made by the body or obtained from sources other than foods and beverages are called nonessential nutrients.[25] They include chemicals like biotin that is produced by gastrointestinal bacteria, cholesterol that is produced by the liver, Vitamin K that is produced by intestinal bacteria, and Vitamin D that is produced by sunlight in the skin.

So, what are the major sources of these nutrients? WHOLE FOODS,[26] Gut bacteria (microbiome) Production, and MOM and DAD!

Whole foods include:

- **Proteins:** meat, dairy, legumes, nuts, seafood, and eggs
- **Carbohydrates:** potatoes, rice, grains, milk, fruit, sugar, vegetables, fruit
- **Fats:** oils, butter, margarine, nuts, seeds, avocados, and olives, meat, and seafood
- **Vitamins:** common vitamins include the water-soluble B group vitamins and Vitamin C; the fat-soluble Vitamins A, D, E and K. Vitamins are commonly found in high levels in plants.
- **Minerals**: (sodium, calcium, iron, iodine, magnesium, potassium, etc.); all nature-derived foods contain some form of minerals.

- **Water** available as a beverage and a component of many foods, especially vegetables and fruits. Water is vital to health.

The Rest of the Story

Among the databases that list food chemistry composition, the U.S. Department of Agriculture (USDA) tracks 188 biochemicals, often called nutritional components. As much as we are trained to think of food as fats, or protein, or carbohydrates, that perception really does an injustice to the complexity and magnificence of the chemistry in food. While our food-regulating organizations track and monitor and, in some ways, regulate these 188 food chemicals, the list represents the tiniest fraction of what actually exists in the food that nature provides. A deeper dive into the food chemistry databases has identified a staggering 26,625 unique chemical compounds present in foods![27]

Consider garlic. Garlic has been a staple food product for much of human history and is key in Mediterranean diets. The USDA identifies 67 nutritional components in raw garlic, with particular notes that garlic is rich in Vitamin B6, selenium, and manganese.[28] That's 67 nutrients, with only three highlighted. The deeper look into the chemical composition of garlic alone has identified a remarkable 2,306 distinct chemical compounds! Well over 2,000 chemical compounds in just garlic alone! Combine the 2,300 chemicals in garlic with the over 1,900 chemicals in the herb sweet basil and another couple of thousand biochemicals in a dose of olive oil and not only do you have a delicious pesto, but you have a vast chemistry-rich pantry from which your body can utilize. The complexity of nature's food is a frontier that is virtually unexplored.[29] There is a new recognition and exploration as to the powerful role that the unacknowledged bioactive chemicals found in food plays in our human function. It is so complex and so unique to the individual who eats these chemistries that our technologies cannot fully comprehend the infinite variations. There is no way to fully supplement what food actually provides (and for the record I utilize and recommend responsible supplementation). For that reason, WE MUST GET THE FOOD AS RIGHT AS POSSIBLE. We must give the body a vast variety of nature-produced foods—nature's chemistries—to help the body have what it needs to function optimally.

The Standard American Diet is profoundly deficient in the critical nutrients necessary for human function, and most people aren't even meeting minimal goals. According to a 2017 report by the Centers for Disease Control and Prevention, just 1:10 adults get the recommended amount of fruits and vegetables.[30] Actually, that deficiency is not a new problem. The deficiency in consumption of plant/nature-based nutrients began as humans transitioned from hunting and gathering to agriculture. This transition affected the strength of our bodies. Skeletal records have noted a lightening of the human skeleton that occurred with the introduction of agriculture 12,000 years ago.[31] The shift to monocrop production and consumption[32] increased food availability and reliability for many and changed how we move, while inadvertently decreasing the variety and availability of vast numbers of unacknowledged nutrients/chemistries.[33,34] Once the family garden started going away in the mid-20th century, the deficiency in these nutritional chemistries became profound.[35]

The Impact

You are so tired. You drag yourself out of bed and never feel energized. You're distracted, anxious, and unable to focus. Maybe an energy drink will get you going. *Nope.* You eat all day long, but somehow, you're still hungry.

Welcome to the modern world of tired and wired. In order to understand what is happening with these chemistries in the cell, consider the revolutionary Ford automobile assembly line. According to Henry Ford, these are the principles of assembly:

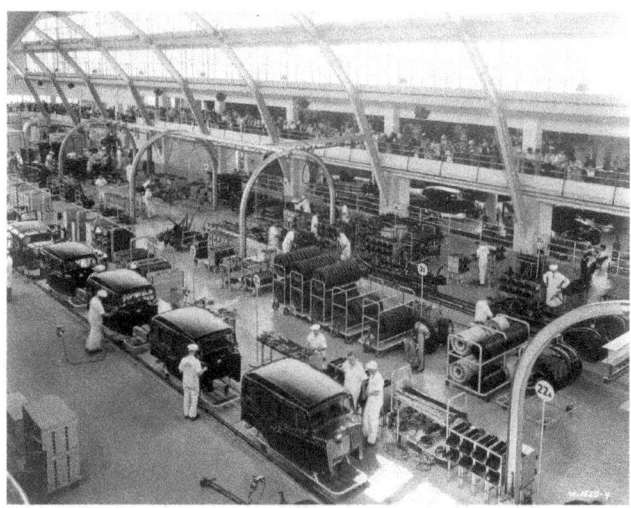

Kaufmann & Fabry Co. "Chevrolet's Automoble Assembly Line—General Motors Building, Century Of Progress." Postcard. 1933. Curt Teich Postcard Archives Digital Collection (Newberry Library). https://collections.carli.illinois.edu/digital/collection/nby_teich/id/415495.

(1) Place the tools and the men in the sequence of the operation so that each component part shall travel the least possible distance while in the process of finishing.

(2) Use work slides or some other form of carrier so that when a workman completes his operation, he drops the part always in the same place—which place must always be the most convenient place to his hand—and if possible, have gravity carry the part to the next workman for his own action.

(3) Use sliding assembling lines by which the parts to be assembled are delivered at convenient distances.[36]

Similar to Ford's factory, our biological machines are made up of complex "chemical assembly lines." Each "line" requires large amounts of "parts" (nutrients) and "workers" (enzymes) to produce the "cars" (energy, muscles, hormones, etc.) necessary for life. Food provides us the "chemical parts and workers" for these metabolic assembly lines and all of the nutrients necessary to produce energy. What happens if not enough "parts" are available or the workers do not show up?

Health Strategy

- Provide your body with enough of what it needs to function. Focus on eating a rich, whole food, plant-focused diet.

Practice

- For one week, write down what you eat for every meal. Don't think of the task as a way to count calories or cut back—think of it as a way to gather information. (Taking a picture with your phone of what you eat is a great, easy way to track.)
- Do you find yourself eating a lot of the same meals? That's okay! Once you have a sense of what you eat in a week, *add* more plant and protein to your menu. The challenge is to eat the rainbow and with each opportunity sneak in a bit more nutrient-dense food.
- Identify deficiencies. Seek out laboratory assessments of your nutrient levels.[37] Ideally your physician or pharmacist will assist you in acquiring such laboratory findings. Many may balk and say "your insurance won't cover it, so I am not going to order it." Do not let that stop you. You are worth the cost of this information, especially if you are not well. The internet allows us to access this valuable information through direct-to-consumer laboratories. (Go to **Ultalabtests.com/DrKathyHealth** to explore laboratory options.)

Some of the nutrients that may be valuable to assess include:

- Vitamin A
- Vitamin C
- Vitamin D
- Vitamin E
- Vitamin K
- Vitamin B1 (thiamine)
- Vitamin B2 (riboflavin)
- Vitamin B3 (niacin)
- Pantothenic acid
- Biotin
- Vitamin B6
- Vitamin B12
- Folate
- Calcium
- Magnesium
- Iron Panel with ferritin
- Sodium
- Zinc, copper
- Phosphorus
- Omega-3 / Omega-6 Index
- Electrolytes (Sodium, Potassium often noted in a Complete Blood Count)
- Pre-albumin and total protein

CHAPTER 4:

Famine of Energy

"Everything is energy and that's all there is to it."

~Darryl Anka

Energy is the ability to move something. For humans and much of life, the energy utilized to beat your heart or hug your child is found in the molecule adenosine triphosphate (ATP).[38] ATP is life's battery pack. Within this tiny molecule is stored the energy that runs life. Many of the "chemical assembly lines" (also known as metabolic pathways) present in living organisms are dedicated to the production of this critical molecule. As THE necessary chemistry of life, much of the body's resources are dedicated to its production. It is estimated that we use our **body weight** in this tiny, precious molecule EVERY DAY![39] Think about that! Every day you make and use your body weight in energy. The proper function of the body relies on adequate ATP production, and you are likely not producing enough. You cannot consume ATP in a pill or through an IV—you must "manufacture" ATP on your own "assembly lines." No ATP, no life.

The energy you need must be produced within your body. Deep within your cells, small organs (organelles) called mitochondria manufacture the energy you need. Mitochondria produce about 90% of the ATP that we need to survive.[40] Just as a car needs fuel, your cells need ATP.

The structure of this small ATP molecule consists of the nitrogenous base adenine, a sugar molecule (ribose), and three serial bonded high-energy phosphate groups.[41]

It is the breaking of the bonds within the phosphate groups that liberates the energy which keeps you warm and breathing. I think of these high-energy bonds in ATP like the strong magnets we played with as kids. ATP enables you to think and solve problems. Interestingly, your brain at rest consumes 20-25% of this energy to function![42] ATP is the energy needed to give birth to and raise your children. This is the energy that beats your heart.

The cells that need the most energy contain the most mitochondria in order to create more ATP.[43] The heart muscle contains an estimated 5,000 mitochondria (cellular factories) per cell![44] It is thought that a single mitochondrion contains an estimated 17,000 assembly lines[45] (electron transport chains or ECT, glycolysis, and Krebs cycles are just a few assembly lines)! Think about that. A single heart cell contains 5,000 mitochondria,[46] each containing 17,000 ECT assembly lines! Each assembly line needs adequate "nuts and bolts" (chemical nutrients), each having to have the worker show up, each doing their job correctly in order to process and produce energy! Consider the amount of ATP and nutrients needed to keep the heart muscle beating and your brain working 24/7, for 70, 80, or 100 years. That is a lot of energy!

Mitochondria house many of your cellular assembly lines, and just like in any factory, there is a bunch of stuff going on in your mitochondrial factories. A key job of mitochondria is to transform those macronutrients[47,48] (protein, carbohydrates, fat) from our diet through the assembly lines into the ATP (energy) needed for life.

The mitochondrial factory can compound $1 of the sugar glucose into an amazing $38 of ATP energy.[49] This is crazy efficient! (There is a bit of debate as to exactly what this number is, but even at the low end of $30 ATP that is a great return on your $1 glucose investment!) For enough energy to be produced, the chemical assembly line must have a *large* number of "chemical parts" available for assembly![50] Basically, a little bit of sugar (fat or protein) plus a large number of micronutrients (vitamins, minerals, oxygen, etc.) and happy/healthy mitochondria equal a large amount of energy.

For most of human history, the chemistry needed for ATP production, also known as life, came from our mother in the womb, the foods we ate, or from the chemistries produced by the bacteria found in our gut. As humans evolved, the foods being consumed, both plant and animal, contained this ratio—small amounts of macronutrients with large amounts of micronutrients. Hunting and gathering ensured that the variety of needed chemistries were available.[51] Precious glucose was always available in small but adequate amounts from green plants and the sun from the process called photosynthesis. And the 13 atoms of oxygen necessary to produce ONE molecule of ATP?[52] Well, that was efficiently delivered to the cells with all of that hunting and gathering (movement) we were tasked with doing to collect those necessary plants/foods! Within the leaves that our ancestors easily grabbed to survive came large amounts of the "nuts and bolts" that our machine would need in order to produce energy.

Without the necessary chemistry, we will not make enough energy. Instead of $38 of ATP, your machine may be forced to survive on $10 or maybe even $2. The difference is a crisis for the cell, and the machine (YOU) will be forced to adapt in order to survive.

The starved cell will send a message to your behavior organ—the brain—and adjustments in your system will be made.[53] The "adjustments" may look like a decrease in temperature, metabolism, mood, energy, cognition—all appropriate actions to match your "demand" to the reduced energy supply.[54] The machine will work to help you survive. For many animals, survival might look like being curled up under a rock, breathing, expending as little precious energy as possible. For us, it may look like being overweight, curled up on the sofa, scrolling social media. For modern humans and for many of my patients, survival often looks like depression, irritability, fatigue, lack of motivation, lower temperature, and, yes, obesity.

The Illusion of Nutrition

If you do not consume (digest and absorb) the chemistry contained in a minimum of 7-10 servings (1 cup uncooked, 1/2 cup cooked) of plants as well as 7-12 servings of protein a day you are likely "misnourished," lack critical micronutrients, and are starving at the cellular level. Changing with each season, hunter-gatherers consumed large varieties of foods every year, each variety containing different chemistries that our machines could harness for function.[55] The largest animals on our planet are vegetarians-eating huge amounts of plants![56] Most of us eat the same 8-10 things, and often those foods do not include vegetables.

We have been led to believe that calories are all that matter and that we are eating too many. That belief is wrong. The calorie conversation is insultingly simplistic and does not take into consideration what makes up the calorie. **It is the chemistry, not the calories, that count!** Food is information. The information and chemistries contained in a 200-calorie chicken breast is very different than the information and chemistries contained in the 200-calorie donut.[57,58] Tragically, this calorie-centric approach of "eat less, exercise more" has made the **famine of chemistry** much worse.[59] It is not uncommon for those of us who have grown up with this approach to "dieting" to find ourselves diagnosed with conditions of nutrient deficiencies such as **osteoporosis, sarcopenia,**[60] **dementia,**[61] **anemia,**[62] **depression,**[63] **accelerated aging, and obesity.**[64] We are starving!

Health Strategy

- Explore and follow a plant-focused Mediterranean lifestyle approach. We must eat a heck of a lot of the right stuff!

Practice

- Audit the foods you routinely eat. Write down (take a picture, track with a digital tool, etc.) the foods that you consume.

How many plants (vegetables, fruits, nuts, legumes, whole grains) did you eat each day? Where do you get your plant chemistry? Go to the produce section at your grocery store and count how many different types of plants are available for purchase. Don't forget to include herbs and the different colors of a specific vegetable.

What patterns did you notice in your food audit?

How do you feel after you eat?

It is important to begin to correlate how the chemistries coming in from our diet are impacting our system. Do you notice changes in your digestion (gas, bloating, reflux, diarrhea, etc.)? Do you notice fatigue?[65] Anxiety?[66] Pain? Energy?[67] Often these impacts are progressive and can occur hours (or even days) after you eat a food. Much like how the body responds to a mosquito bite, the body begins to slowly react after that bite. Over the next two or three days the bite area swells and itches in response, gradually resolving and going back to normal.[68] For many, the body reacts in a similar way with one "bite" of wheat/gluten or dairy.[69] The body "swells" and reacts, except instead of resolving in two or three days, we eat that triggering food again in three hours![70] Many of us know we react to pollens and grass, but do not consider our reactions to the grasses we consume by mouth (corn and wheat are in the grass family). Recognizing and avoiding these reactions can transform your life!

Consider tracking your blood glucose with continuous blood glucose monitoring (CGM).[71] This is a powerful way to monitor over a 24-hour period the impact of diet and stress on blood sugar levels and more importantly begin to correlate these levels to how you feel. (Go to **drkathysays.com/cgm** for more information.)

CHAPTER 5:

Famine of the Gut

"Gut health is the key to overall health."

~Kris Carr

If you eat a perfect diet and take the best supplements but your gut doesn't absorb them, did you actually eat it? The answer is a big NO. For our cells to get what they need, the body must be able to take in the correct nutrients, process and absorb these chemicals, and keep the bad chemistry (or invaders) out! In this section we will cover one of the biggest contributors to obesity and modern disease: the damaged gut.

We are what we eat, absorb, and utilize. Digestion starts from the minute we start thinking about food. When we think about, acquire, or prepare food, our body starts making the chemistry needed to receive the food, break it down, absorb it, and use it. Once we see, smell, or even think about food, you will begin to salivate (chemical breakdown). Ideally, you will prepare (chop, mix, cook), take in, and chew food (mechanical breakdown), swallowing it down into a stomach that's full of hydrochloric acid.

It is crazy to think each of us has a bowl of battery acid in the middle of our bodies. Imagine what happens when you place hydrochloric acid on your skin. OUCH! The result is burning and blistering. Well, that is exactly what's happening when food enters a stomach full of acid. The stomach is a muscular organ perfectly designed to contain large amounts of acid to churn and process our food. A thick layer of mucus protects the stomach from damage by its contents.[72]

Down from our mouth and at the end of our esophagus/throat is a muscular gate, the lower esophageal sphincter (LES)[73] that allows food into the stomach and keeps the acid from escaping up into our more delicate, unprotected throats.[74]

How well the LES works to keep the acid where it belongs depends at least in part on how much acid is in the stomach. If you have a lot of acid, your LES will be like a tight, clamped-down gate. If you have a little acid, your LES will be like a lazy, leaky gate.[75] Also important to a tight LES are the minerals involved in muscle contraction—magnesium and calcium. Low amounts of these minerals may lead to weakened muscular contractions.[76] What leads to low amounts of minerals you might ask? Low stomach acid! Magnesium, calcium, iron, zinc are literally rocks that must be transformed into an absorbable form with the chemical reactions occurring in a bath of acid.[77] Even if we consume enough of those essential minerals from our diet (which most of us do not), a stomach with low acid will not allow for their optimal absorption.

Alcohol, coffee, chocolate, tomatoes, and spicy foods can also loosen this gate, allowing the acid to sneak upward.[78] OUCH!

Acid is important.

The gut must figure out how to keep the stuff coming into the body from killing you. One of the key roles stomach acid plays in your health is to sterilize the food you eat and to prevent harmful bacteria and parasites from entering the gastrointestinal (GI) tract and then into your bloodstream.

A stomach low in acid might lead to an overgrowth of bacteria in areas of the body where there should be little. Normally, our bacterial friends live and work in the lower part of the digestive tract, the large intestine. An overgrowth of bacteria just outside of the stomach (in the small intestine) due to this lack of suppression by the acid can result in severe bloating, especially when one eats sugar or carbohydrates(breads, pasta, cereals, potatoes, soda, etc.).[79]

With high bacterial overgrowth in the upper digestive tract, often the food (nutrients) you eat may never get to you. The bacteria get first dibs on all of the good stuff. They are consuming much of the nutrition taken in with your meal, thus contributing to our cellular starvation.

If you think frequent bloating may apply to you, I suggest you look into Small Intestinal Bacterial Overgrowth (SIBO)[80] and specifically the information from my friend and mentor Elizabeth Lipski's PhD book *Digestive Wellness*. More importantly and immediately, lowering your carbohydrate and sugar intake will give quick relief to the bloating.

A second major role of acid in the stomach is in the transformation of food into absorbable units of chemistry that can be utilized by the body. Macro- and micronutrients are the "nuts and bolts ingredients" critical for life. These chemistries are dependent on acid transformation within the stomach for absorption later in the intestines and into the bloodstream and ultimately into the cell to be utilized. No–or–low acid often results in decreased nutrient absorption and thus the functional starvation at the cellular level.

Take, for example, the mineral iron. By mass, iron is the most common element on the earth.[81] Iron is an essential element for almost all living organisms.[82] Strong and heavy, it is hard to imagine this rock being critical for human life, but it is. Iron has the unique and valuable chemical ability to attract, carry, and release other chemicals. Because of that function, the body relies on iron for the production of blood, the transportation of oxygen throughout the body, production of deoxyribonucleic acid (DNA), and for cellular respiration (ATP production) in the mitochondria (electron transport).[83] Iron is *really* important to the body's function. Without adequate acid in the stomach, the iron coming in from the diet will not be converted into an absorbable form. The rock will pass through the gut never to be absorbed into the bloodstream.

It is just a bit *IRON*ic that the most common element on earth makes up the most common human nutrient deficiency. Research suggests that as much as 80%[84] of people in the world don't have enough iron in their bodies (iron deficient). It also suggests that as much as 30% of people have anemia[85] (not enough red blood cells) due to prolonged iron deficiency. Even mild and moderate forms of iron deficiency can affect cognitive development, the immune system, and our work capacity. Many physicians rarely assess iron status, and if they do, it is only after the deficiency is severe enough to cause anemia. One could have iron deficiency for a decade (latent iron deficiency) before the body can finally no longer adjust, which is when anemia may show up.

Unimaginable fatigue, weakness, shortness of breath, headaches, anxiety, weight gain, and rapid heartbeat are potential symptoms of low iron often attributed to something else. Lack of iron (all of the minerals, really) is a real crisis for the body, resulting in appropriate adaptations for survival. Slower metabolism, reduced thyroid function, fatigue, depression, reduced temperature, and, yes, weight gain might just be the only ways your body can survive without iron's critical chemistry. No acid, no iron. No iron, no oxygen.[86] No oxygen, no energy.[87]

If you have chronic issues with weight or energy, it is important to assess iron/ferritin levels before beginning any non-food supplementation.[88] The only thing worse than too little iron, is too much! Until you are told you have too much iron, eat your liver. ☺

When protein-rich foods enter the stomach, they are greeted by a mixture of hydrochloric acid and the enzyme pepsin. The acidic environment breaks up (denatures) proteins within food. Pepsin cuts proteins into smaller proteins and then into their basic building blocks: amino acids. The body will then absorb these building blocks and assemble them into needed tissues—new muscles, new bone, new brain tissue, new blood. No stomach acid, no amino acids, no new tissue.[89,90]

Adequate protein intake **and** absorption are absolutely necessary for maintaining muscle and metabolism[91,92] throughout life and especially as we age. Low protein absorption leads to low muscle mass. Low muscle mass leads to a lowered metabolic rate (fewer mitochondria) and lowered ATP production.[93] Remember, no ATP, no life. Sarcopenia (low muscle), low energy, and obesity become the new normal. Sound familiar?

The famine of chemistry is ultimately about lacking enough critical chemicals to optimally run our human machine. Critically, low acid leads to low protein, inadequate B-vitamins, and reduced minerals in the bloodstream, which can lead to low muscle mass, low cellular function (low metabolism), and ultimately a body that must adapt to survive.[94,95]

Health Strategy
- Support your gut in working optimally.

Practice
- Assess your gut function.
- Complete the Digestive Assessment (https://innovativehealing.com)

How often do you have gas? Bloating? Constipation? Heartburn? Diarrhea? How often do you find yourself reaching for antacids? These are clues!

It is common that we normalize or suppress (medicate) abnormal gut function in our society. It is not particularly acceptable that we discuss our bowel functions at the dinner table, with our friends, or even with our physician. Symptoms that you have tolerated, even normalized for years—constipation, running to the bathroom after a meal—may be clues to poor function and likely could be contributing to your famines.

Consider adding probiotic-rich foods to your grocery list.[96] Such foods can include yogurt, sauerkraut, kimchi, kombucha, pickles, and kefir.

While you're at it, consider adding polyphenols-rich foods into your diet.[97] These molecules feed the good microbes in your gut. Some good sources of polyphenols include red grapes, wine made from those same grapes, green tea, onions, blueberries, broccoli, and dark chocolate. Eat Plants!!

CHAPTER 6:
Famine of Stomach Acid

"The road to health is paved with good intestines."

~Sherry A. Rogers

Now that you know the importance of good stomach acid, what would be the cause of too little stomach acid? Surprisingly, aging is often cited as a common reason for low production of stomach acid.[98] Aging is often used as a too convenient explanation of many of our ailments. I think of aging as being the result of chronic deficiency. Low dietary intake (due to culture, availability, and preferences) and increased dietary need (high carbohydrate diet, increased excretion from medications, and stress) lead to the body's not having enough chemistry to work well. The body must have adequate B-vitamins in order for the stomach to make needed acid. Low stomach acid due to aging is more likely to be the result of a diet low in the B-vitamins needed to produce acid and reduces the acid available to process and absorb the B-vitamins. It's a nasty, vicious circle! Without stomach acid, the body will not properly break down proteins or absorb these other critical chemistries, thus increasing the rate of aging and the risks of diseases of malnutrition—sarcopenia,[99] iron deficiency anemia,[100] B-12 deficiency,[101] osteoporosis,[102] etc.

Rather than from aging, a much bigger contributor to low gastric acid comes again from the modern pharmaceutical industry. Many medications either intentionally or unintentionally reduce stomach acid production. Drugs that have anticholinergics effects[103] (drying effects) are widely used for a variety of conditions and are easily available over the counter in the form of antihistamines.[104] The short-term use of these medications can be lifesaving. The long-term use can and does seem to have severely negative effects that may in part be a result of the lack of acid and subsequent lack of nutrient absorption.

Acid-blocking drugs were developed in the mid-20th century as a solution to life-threatening peptic ulcer disease. For decades, surgeons were taught and believed that peptic ulcer disease was caused by acid, and treatments were focused on the elimination of acid through surgery or acid-reducing drug therapies. The 1970s brought the research and development of two classes of acid-suppressing drugs, the Histamine-2 antagonists (H2 blockers) and the proton-pump inhibitors (PPIs), notably Cimetidine, 1976, and Omeprazole, 1989.[105] The newer approach, using PPIs, was quickly shown to be clinically superior to the H2 blockers at reducing acid. Proton-pump inhibitors and H2 blockers suppress acid in two very different ways. PPIs are the on/off switch of acid production; H2s are the volume switch. While both will produce relief to the patient suffering from reflux and ulcers, there seems to be very different long-term consequences to the body in their use. Recent studies have correlated long-term PPI use with dementia, stroke, osteoporosis, kidney failure, early death, and, yes, obesity.[106]

Omeprazole (Losec/Prilosec) became the world's biggest selling pharmaceutical ever, and to date, hundreds of millions of patients have been treated worldwide.[107] Over-the-counter availability to these acid-reducing therapies has provided global access to individuals seeking relief without a consultation with a medical professional. What was initially developed to treat life-threatening peptic ulcers, soon became the preferred remedy for too many chili dogs or eating too late—the uncomfortable but seldom life-threatening heartburn or gastric-esophageal reflux symptoms. With each dose we unknowingly reduce the acid needed to digest and absorb critical nutrients. In essence, we starve the cell, contributing to our Modern Famine.[108]

Common Acid Issues

Acid chemically breaks down or transforms much of what it touches. Gastroesophageal Reflux Disease (GERD), commonly known as acid reflux,[109] has kept many a physician very busy. Much of our gut discomfort with GERD comes from this balanced system being disrupted—the overproduction of acid due to bacteria or stress, a diet and lifestyle that does not support good digestion, or acid that just does not stay where it belongs due to physical impairment. Decreased mucus to protect the stomach from medications may also weaken the stomach's protection.[110]

Modern humans are plagued with gut issues and low absorption of nutrients. Much of on what and how we survive within our modern life could damage the body, and the body in its wisdom often protects us by how it responds. Our crazy modern culture has created the perfect conditions for this digestive chaos.

It is no wonder these classes of acid-blocking drugs have become so widely used. They are very effective in reducing the immediate pain caused by the acid. Their use, and arguably overuse, though, has been at a tremendous cost to our health: cellular starvation and a machine that lacks the basic chemistry to work.

Chronic acid in the esophagus can lead to scarring and potentially esophageal cancer—very serious conditions. For some individuals/situations, pharmaceutical intervention may always be a necessary tool. These gastric aids should be only used after supporting a healthy digestive system and a healthy gut. Ask yourself: Why is my acid not staying where it is supposed to? Why do I have gas? Why do I have reflux? What can I do to have a healthy and happy stomach?

Health Strategy

- Optimize your digestive function.

Practice

- Audit what medications you take and their effects on your stomach acid/digestion. If you are taking an acid-blocking medication in the PPI (omeprazole, etc.) class,[111] work with your doctor and pharmacist to transition to a more moderate acid suppressor, H2 blocker (Pepcid), or, better yet, to support your gut in not needing those medications.
- Use your health journal to write down how your gut works with the different foods you eat. Notice the foods that trigger discomfort or a noticeable body response. Notice the foods that sooth or support your digestion.
- Audit the carbohydrates in your life! Begin to reduce the amount of sugar in your diet. All carbohydrates ultimately break down into sugar. Focus on getting your carbohydrates from vegetables and fruits. What do you notice?
- Consider adding "acid" to your meals in the form of vinegars (acetic acids) or from citrus fruits (lemons, limes, oranges, etc.). Beginning your meal with a wonderful vinaigrette salad can be a lovely way to enhance the digestion of your meal.

A TRILLION Friends

It is thought that only 10% of the DNA (genetic material) in a human body is actually human.[112]

I was shocked and puzzled when I first heard that statistic. My next thought was, "What is the other 90% made of?!"

Within our gut (throughout the body, really) is a universe of bacterial, mitochondrial, fungal, and viral DNA. It is estimated that for every one human gene, there is may be 100-150 non-human genes present within this universe![113] So, I ask you: Are we hosting them, or are they hosting us? We are being hosted by an ecosystem of (mostly) friendly bacteria, viruses, fungus, yeast-microbes, or microbiota that actually live and work within our bodies. They run the show. More than a thousand bacterial species and nine million unique microbial genes[114,115] are estimated to be associated with a healthy human body, according to the National Institute of Health's National Human Genome Research Institute.

Most of the microbes within our system do not cause disease—quite the contrary. We actually rely on microbes to perform critical functions we cannot ourselves perform. Microbes, also sometimes termed probiotics, live their lives within our systems, digest foods, synthesize vitamins, metabolize drugs, detoxify carcinogens, stimulate renewal of cells in the gut lining, and activate and support the immune system. They also keep "bad" bacteria under control with a bit of healthy competition. There are beneficial bacteria systems on our skin, in our lungs, through our urinary tract, and even in our brain.[116] We are just beginning to comprehend the vital contribution of our microbial hosts to our human function and dysfunction.

It is estimated that these microbes produce an estimated 25%+ (low estimate) of the critical chemistries needed for the host cells (us) to function.[117] The chemicals produced by the bacteria in our guts are termed "postbiotics" and are critical for optimal body function and in some cases are sources of dysfunction.[118] What happens if this bacterial army are not fed well or are damaged in some way? Well, they cannot do their job. When they are not well, we (the host) are not well due to a deficiency in the nutrients that healthy bacteria would produce—hence, contributing to our Modern Famine.

The gut bacteria love fiber, they love plants! The foods that bacteria eat are generally termed "prebiotics." More specifically, prebiotics are defined as substrate that is selectively utilized by host microorganisms conferring a health benefit.[119] Indeed, what we need to eat is often not primarily for us alone! There is value in thinking about what we eat as creating a rich garden in which our microbial friends can flourish. Plants have much of what our beneficial bacteria, "the good bacteria," need to produce the critical chemistries for our systems. Our current culture has made life for our gut bacteria very difficult.

Complicating poor nutrition further, the 1970s brought about the development of pesticides like the weed-killer glyphosate (also known as Roundup). It has been found to be carcinogenic to humans, and it is catastrophic for our bacterial friends.[120] The same way that pesticides and herbicides destroy bugs and weeds in the fields, they are destroying the bacteria that take care of our human machine.[121]

At about the same time began the development and explosion of the use of medicinal antibacterials. Antibiotics, including penicillin, sulfonamides, and antibacterial lotions, became widely accessible and widely used in both human and veterinary medicine.[122]

Antibiotics, including antibacterials in cleaning products, toothpastes, as well as antibiotics used in the production of our food, ultimately and profoundly impact our bacterial balance. These antibacterial agents are indiscriminate in their killing of bacteria. Our efforts to kill "bad" bacteria inadvertently kill the "good" or beneficial bacteria! Low quantities of beneficial bacteria as well as elevated levels of pathogenic bacteria are fueling the rise in some of the diseases plaguing our modern societies. The overuse of these at times life-saving antibiotics have created unforeseen challenges.

This overzealous use of antibacterial agents has inadvertently created a very disrupted and damaged microbial universe. We are just beginning to recognize the profound impact the practice has had on our health.[123]

With regard to antibiotics and obesity, the research is clear.

As researchers looked into the relationship of antibiotic use in childhood and the development of obesity later in life, one study asked, "What are we doing to our children?"[124] The researchers clearly correlated the disruption of our microbiome due to antibiotic use to the creation of the biological conditions contributing to societal obesity.[125]

What bacteria we have in our system, where they live, what friends they have (probiotics), what they have to eat (prebiotics), and in what environment they find themselves are as important as if we were asking those questions for ourselves, possibly more so. Just one round of antibiotics can disrupt the "bacterial balance" for two years![126]

Much like a tornado ripping through a community or a bomb going off, the destruction to the microbiome universe with these environmental toxins is profound. Each exposure to antibiotics or pesticides/herbicides forever changes the landscape of life. The bacteria that work, play, and live in our systems are fighting to survive! Our bacteria's environment, their "culture," the medium on which they grow, has been enormously challenged over the last 100 years, and they (and us) are not doing well.

Health Strategy

- Support your microbiome! Create a healthy, robust bacterial army!

Practice

- Minimize pesticide-laden food. Buy and eat organic, hormone-free produce when possible. (Why we have to pay

more for non-poisoned food is a pet-peeve of mine and likely a topic left to a later book!)
- Grow your own food. (Extra credit!)
- Wash all produce very well before eating.
- Encourage your body to excrete toxins through good elimination! (Pee, drink water; poop, veggies/protein; sweat, exercise; breathe, movement!)
- Meet with a pharmacist to have a complete medication/vitamin review.
- Add to your timeline/health journal how many rounds of antibiotics you have had in your lifetime. Last five years? Last six months?
- What effects have you seen in your health following antibiotic use?
- What do you feed your microbiome? How many servings of plant (vegetables, legumes, nuts, fruit, etc.) have you consumed in the last 24 hours? 7 days? 30 days?
- Calculate the amount of fiber consumed daily for a week.
- Do you buy and eat organic produce?
- Do you use antibacterial soaps?
- Add probiotic-rich food to your diet! Fermented vegetables and dairy can be a great way to support a healthy gut.

Don't stress about your answers here. Instead, use them to become more aware of your habits and identify ways you can make small, easy changes. You don't have to go out and buy a farm, but maybe you can plant a small garden or grow some herbs in your windowsill. Maybe you can swap out some of your regular produce for organic. Focus where you can. Just increasing your plant/fiber consumption toward that 7-10 servings a day will have tremendous positive impacts on the health of you and your bacterial friends.

Leaky Gut

Once food has passed the acid bath of the stomach, digestion continues to the small intestines and absorption picks up. Many added chemical helpers known as enzymes are produced and added to the food-acid mix. Enzymes enhance the breakdown of food, readying nutrients for absorption.[127] The gut is very careful what it allows into the bloodstream.[128] The intestinal lining is one cell thick[129] and contains small portals for absorption referred to as "tight junctions."[130] These small portals are tasked with allowing in the good (nutrients) and keeping out the bad (toxins and bacteria). Allowing bacteria or toxins into the bloodstream could be fatal.

Sometimes the body opens wide these portals in an effort to "let more in." During periods of high demand or high stress, the body risks being less discerning by opening up the gates and ushering in more fuel. Toxins, medications, or antibacterials can have a damaging effect on these tight junctions as well.[131] Unfortunately, when the "tight junctions" are not tight, things get into the bloodstream that ideally should not be there. The term popularly used to describe this is "leaky gut," which is a generalized term describing increased intestinal permeability.[132]

When the gut is "leaky," it allows substances to be absorbed into the bloodstream that may not otherwise be allowed.[133] The research in this field is recent and exciting. In a groundbreaking paper, Dr. Alessio Fasano discussed increased intestinal permeability and its impact on our health.

"Genetic predisposition, mis-communication between innate and adaptive immunity, exposure to environmental triggers, and loss of intestinal barrier function secondary to the activation of the zonulin (a protein that increases the permeability of the gut)[134] pathway by food-derived environmental triggers or changes in gut microbiota, all seem to be key ingredients involved in the pathogenesis of inflammation, autoimmunity, and cancer."[135]

Basically, once the gut leaks and allows stuff into the bloodstream, the body's SWAT team is called in. The immune system is activated to attack these chemical threats—the poorly digested, big chunks of "stuff" (proteins, toxins, polysaccharides, etc.) from the low acid stomach or from bacteria that survived and made it through the big leaky gates into the bloodstream. Unfortunately, there is often collateral damage in the "SWAT" team attack.

In a process described by the term "molecular mimicry," the immune system attacks everything that resembles the invading protein.[136] Imagine you lived at the address 130 S. Main Street. The postman, instead of just delivering your mail to 130 S. Main, incorrectly decides to deliver it to 130 S. Elm or 130 S. Maple. In the case of molecular mimicry, the immune system attacks the undigested protein sequence (130) that look like the offending bacteria as well as all of the other similarly looking proteins in the body...130 S. Thyroid (Hashimoto's[137]), 130 S. Cartilage (Rheumatoid Arthritis[138]), or 130 S. Pancreas (Type 1 Diabetes[139]). Ideally, you have fully digested your proteins down to their individual numbers (amino acids). The immune system will not react to the 1 or the 3 or the 0 individually. But when the combination (130) is presented, the immune system sees this as a threat and attacks. Poor digestion and a leaky gut allow into the bloodstream foreign substances triggering an appropriate immune response (SWAT team). Inadvertently, you the host are attacked in the process. The aftermath looks like pain, inflammation, depression, obesity, and much of the autoimmune epidemic[140] we are seeing today.

What would cause a gut to leak? Modern life. As Dr. Fasano commented, "genetic predisposition, environmental triggers and loss of intestinal barrier function" are key causes.[141]

More specifically, the culprits include modern medications (antibiotics, acid blockers, non-steroidal anti-inflammatories), chronic high stress (cortisol), environmental triggers (processed foods, toxins, pathogens, alcohol, smoking, heavy metals, etc.), and modern eating habits.

Our modern Western culture has created chaos and has profoundly disrupted our delicate gut/body/environment balance. With regard to obesity, the gut cannot successfully absorb the necessary chemicals for adequate metabolic function. Big challenge. The chemicals that do make it into the bloodstream can trigger an all-out attack of the immune system. Bigger challenge. Current research suggests that this runaway immune system could indeed be a contributor to obesity.[142,143]

Does any of this seem familiar? Reflux, diarrhea, constipation, inflammation, weight gain, crazy hunger, fatigue, pain, medication, more weight gain, hunger, inflammation, and pain. A truly vicious circle.

For many, it is a situation that has taken years to create or for some begun the day they were born (maybe even before that). Creating a new reality is possible. The body has an amazing ability to heal, to change. We must create new conditions for the body to function within. When we do that, we will get new results.

Health Strategy

- Heal your gut! Optimize gut function.

Practice

- On your timeline, identify events where your body may have been under increased demands or increased stress. You already have noted those times with antibiotic use, but do not forget pregnancy, college, marriage, car accidents, deaths. Those are very demanding times.
- Add to your health journal an audit of pain and inflammation. When do you hurt? Do you swell? What triggers pain? Keep track of how much and what kind of

food and drink you consume throughout the day. It can also be helpful to keep track of whom you were with and what mood you were in while eating those foods.
- Again, audit your carbohydrate intake. Calculate your net carbohydrates by taking the total carbohydrates from your food and subtracting the total fiber within the meal.

CARB COUNTING 101

TOTAL CARBOHYDRATES
− TOTAL FIBER
NET CARBOHYDRATES

https://nutritiondata.self.com

DrKathy Health, LLC

Nutrition Facts
Serving Size 1 Medium Apple (182g / 6.4oz)

Amount Per Serving	
Calories 95	Calories from Fat 3

	% Daily Value*
Total Fat 0g	1%
Saturated Fat 2g	0%
Trans Fat 0g	
Cholesterol 0mg	0%
Sodium 2mg	0%
Total Carbohydrate 25g	8%
Dietary Fiber 4g	17%
Sugars 19g	
Protein 0g	

| Vitamin A 2% | • | Vitamin C 14% |
| Calcium 1% | • | Iron 1% |

*Percent Daily Values are based on a 2,000 calorie diet. Your daily values may be higher or lower depending on your calorie needs.

	Calories	2,000	2,500
Total Fat	Less than	65g	50g
Sat Fat	Less than	20g	25g
Cholesterol	Less than	300mg	300mg
Sodium	Less than	2,400mg	2,400mg
Total Carbohydrate		300mg	375mg
Dietary Fiber		25g	30g

- Are you routinely eating foods that are produced with pesticides or herbicides?
- Listen to and document what your body is telling you. Look to your timeline to begin to correlate external inputs (life, trauma, illness, medications, foods, etc.) to your body's response. If you eat bread, do you have bloating and gas? If you drink a soda, do you notice pain, anxiety or loss of energy? Remember that you are the only you. Only you can fully understand your unique machine. Mapping those circumstances will give you (and your health team) tremendous clues for healing.

CHAPTER 7:
Famine of Chemistry

*"The greatest medicine of all is teaching
people how not to need it."*

~Hippocrates

So, what happens if the body does not have enough chemistry to work? Think of it like baking a cake without all the ingredients. Nutrients provide nourishment essential for growth and the maintenance of life. They are the nuts, bolts, and workers for your chemical assembly lines. Think food, oxygen, and water.

Oxygen is arguably ***the*** essential nutrient.[144] That energy currency we spoke of earlier, ATP, requires a remarkable 13 atoms of oxygen to be made! No oxygen, no ATP, no life. Imagine the body's desperation in not having enough oxygen. The body freaks out. The body does anything and everything to adapt and survive this crisis and sometimes it's not pretty. Diseases of low oxygen (such as emphysema, asthma, COPD, heart disease, and sleep apnea) are particularly difficult to experience, not to mention observe. The body's adaptive symptoms of insomnia, fear, and anxiety[145] are severe and unrelenting. A necessary increase of heart rate and blood pressure may occur to increase delivery of that precious cargo to hungry cells. A ridiculously high amount of the diseases being treated today have a correlation to low oxygen.[146] Obesity represents a reduced metabolic need and is just one symptom of many survival strategies the body may used to have you survive low oxygenation. Add to this fatigue, depression, hypertension, osteoporosis, irritability—all appropriate (and too common) symptoms of too little cellular oxygen. The body does whatever it takes to keep you alive.

When the body does not have enough chemistry to work, it is tasked with prioritizing where precious resources must go. Renowned biochemist Dr. Bruce Ames has discussed this issue in his Triage Theory.[147] Also referred to as the Triage Theory of Aging, Dr. Ames and colleagues suggest that some functions of micronutrients (the approximately 40 essential vitamins, minerals, fatty acids, and amino acids) are restricted during shortage and that the functions required for short-term survival take precedence over those that are less essential.[148]

Basically, the body must use the limited chemicals (nutrients) available to keep you alive ***now***, not worrying about down the road, your reproduction, or your living along time. Like the importance of oxygen, consider another important nutrient, Vitamin K.[149] When you are tremendously deficient, the body must decide the most critical place to put that critical chemistry in order for you to survive. Dr. Ames and his colleagues suggest that the body will prioritize this Vitamin K to the urgent action of blood clotting so that you do not bleed to death. This reallocation will be at the expense of other important but less urgent Vitamin K actions of bone and blood vessel repair, ultimately contributing to diseases of aging, osteoporosis or bone loss, and arterial calcification (heart disease).

Ditto for iron. Not enough iron? The body is going to send its precious resources to the red blood cells so it can bind and circulate oxygen. Needless to say, getting that oxygen to the cell is pretty important. But as a result, less iron will be available for mitochondria's iron to make ATP/energy (fatigue), to make new DNA, or to make necessary hormones. There also will be less iron for your thyroid function and as a result a lowered metabolism. Being tired or depressed because of low iron (or any low nutrient for that matter) is a great survival strategy because you will use less oxygen. You will survive. But for how long?

The body will prioritize short-term survival at the expense of the long-term survival. I often think of it like a small city government: if the economy is good, and there are lots of taxes coming in, all the potholes in the roads will be fixed; if there is a crisis and fewer tax dollars are available, all the resources go to police and fire. Critical functions are the priority. To the body, it is not critical that you be thin, happy, or energetic. Its priority is what does the body have to do to keep you breathing? What does it have to do to keep you warm? Sometimes survival looks a lot like obesity, depression, anxiety, and irritability. The body is not concerned with our modern-day version of appearance and success. It is concerned with your primitive survival. It is estimated that up to 55% of women may be deficient in iron! And that is just one of many critical nutrients!

So, what does being "nutrient deficient" look like, you ask? MODERN LIFE! Fatigue, obesity, infertility, brain fog, depression...yes. The following chart looks at the different stages of nutrient deficiency. Early signs of nutrient deficiency exhibit few symptoms and may only clinically be noted with in-depth blood work. Stages 1 and 2 of nutrient deficiency may only be detected with analysis through blood or urine.[150] It is the rare physician who will order laboratory tests to look for nutrient deficiencies. It is rarer that insurance will pay for nutrient deficiency testing! Both are wrong to neglect these fundamental assessments in order to proactively head off the diseases that are just around the corner. For many, Stage 3 nutrient deficiency is just the *first* time that physical symptoms—lack of energy, malaise, loss of appetite, and insomnia—are noticed. Stage 3 nutrient deficiency[151] is defined as a reduced secretion of micronutrient-dependent enzymes or hormones. Up to that advanced point, the body has adapted and adjusted to keep going. That late realization is what I see in my pharmacy every day. There is a plague of fatigue, insomnia and chronic disease in our modern life.[152,153] What if nutrient deficiency is the underlying cause?

STAGE	ETIOLOGY	EVIDENCE
	The sub-clinical stages of marginal micronutrient deficiency	
STAGE 1	Depletion of vitamin stores	Measurement of vitamin/mineral levels in blood or tissues
STAGE 2	Non-specific biochemical adaptation	Decreased excretion of metabolites in the urine
STAGE 3	Secretion of micronutrient dependent enzymes or hormones reduced	First physical signs; lack of energy, malaise, loss of appetitie, insomnia
STAGE 4	Reversible impairment of metabolic pathways and cellular function	Morphological, metabolic or functional disturbances
STAGE 5	Irreversible tissue damage	Clinical signs of micronutrient deficiency

Concept of borderline vitamin deficiencies, IntJ Vitam Nutr Res Suppl, 1985;27:61-73.

Why are you nutrient deficient? How did you get so starved of these essential nutrients?

Deficiency has several possible reasons and may be the result of:

- **Lack of consumption** (cultural, quality, and economic availability of nutrients)
- **Reduced absorption** (diminished gut function)
- **Increased requirement** (increased metabolic need, i.e., sugar-rich diet needing more B-vitamins and ATP to process, increased metabolic demand on body due to stress, toxins, medications, trauma, lack of recovery, etc.)
- **Increased loss** (due to medications, disease, or genetics)

Lack of Consumption

Not getting enough "food" is not something we would consider in Western society, especially when looking around and seeing that almost 75% of us are overweight or obese. Contrary to appearances, the reality is that we live in a society that is very mis-nourished, if not malnourished. We have lots of "food-like substances" and very little of the nutrition (chemistry) our bodies need for function. This "illusion of nutrition" is the reason that medicine overlooks and will not assess nutrient deficiency. Physicians often look at their obese patients and assume they eat too much and that deficiencies in nutrients cannot be possible. As you can tell at this point in this book, I believe they could not be more clinically misguided.

Currently, our standard American diet looks like this:

- 63% of calories come from refined and processed foods (e.g., soft drinks, packaged snacks like potato chips, packaged desserts, etc.)
- 25% of calories come from animal-based foods
- 12% of calories come from plant-based foods

Unfortunately, half of the plant-based calories (6%) come from French fries; only 6% are coming from nutrient-dense plants in the form of fruits, vegetables, whole grains, nuts, and seeds.[154]

You know the diet. Sugary cereals, pop tarts, bagels and juice for breakfast; chicken nuggets, burgers, French fries and soda for lunch; and pizza or pasta for dinner. Cookies, chips, and sweet, caffeinated drinks in between. Unfortunately, the children growing up who have been conditioned to these fast foods have become adults who want and eat larger portions of these "kid's meals" as indicated by the most successful restaurants of the day.[155]

What our culture identifies and encourages as food is now predominantly based on Wall Street's profitability, not the biochemistry (plants and protein) that your body needs to function. Highly processed—highly profitable—food-like substances are EVERYWHERE! Easily and cheaply obtained, easy to eat. I jokingly say that people often bring me donuts, but they almost never bring me broccoli. Plants do not show up easily in our culture or in our day. The results are staggering.

The results of this diet look like this:

- Roughly half of American adults have one or more chronic diseases related to poor diet and inactivity
- Preventable diseases include cardiovascular disease, hypertension, Type 2 diabetes, and some cancers
- More than two-thirds of American adults are overweight or obese
- Nearly one-third of children are overweight or obese
- Increased male and female infertility[156]
- Chronic diseases disproportionately affect low-income/low-resource communities
- Focus on disease treatment rather than on prevention increases and strains health care costs and reduces overall health[157]

The Standard American Diet—or more accurately the Standard American Culture (SAD/SAC)—sadly represents a culturally sponsored mis-nourishment and unfortunately gives us the "illusion of nutrition."

Cooking? What's cooking?

Approximately 63% of all calories consumed in America come from refined or processed foods and is the driver of our current health crisis! Food processing involves the physical, biological, and chemical processes that occur after foods are separated from nature and before they are consumed or used in the preparation of dishes and meals. The apple that has fallen from the tree and was washed before eating has had a bit of processing. Your cutting, tossing, cooking, and chewing is food processing. A change in the food chemistry occurs with each amount of processing and often results in a decrease in the chemistries present in the foods. It is important to understand and critique how the food in our life has been processed. Our lives could depend on it.

Group 1-Unprocessed or Minimally Processed Foods

Unprocessed or natural foods are obtained directly from plants or animals and do not undergo any alteration following their removal from nature. Minimally processed foods are natural foods that have been submitted to cleaning, removal of inedible or unwanted parts, fractioning, grinding, drying, fermentation, pasteurization, cooling, freezing, or other processes that may subtract part of the food but which do not add oils, fats, sugar, salt, or other substances to the original food.[158] *We should consume most of our foods from THIS category!*

Group 2-Processed Culinary Ingredients

Processed culinary ingredients are products extracted from natural foods or from nature by processes such as pressing, grinding, crushing, pulverizing, and refining. They are used in homes and restaurants to season and cook food, and thus create varied and delicious dishes and meals of all types, including broths and soups, salads, pies, breads, cakes, sweets, and preserves. This is cooking! Critical to your health is **your** processing Group 1 through cooking.

Group 3-Processed Foods ("Franken Foods")

There is a very big difference between your "processing" (a.k.a., cooking) your food and Wall Street processing your food. You care about your health, they don't. Group 3 processed food is where the toxic chaos begins.

Processed foods are products manufactured by industry with the use of salt, sugar, oil, or other substances (Group 2) added to natural or minimally processed foods (Group 1) to preserve or to make them more palatable and desirable. They are derived directly from foods and are recognized as versions of the original foods. They are usually consumed as a part of or as a side dish in culinary preparations made using natural or minimally processed foods. Most processed foods have two or three ingredients. In order for these products to be profitable, large amounts of salt, sugars, or oils often are added to enhance flavor or extend shelf life. Beyond their addictive nature, these added chemistries are making us sick.[159] A good rule of thumb is to only eat foods with salt and sugar where you personally added these ingredients. Avoid trusting your food and your health to manufacturers who are tasked with shareholder profits over the health of the consumer.

Group 4-Ultra-Processed Foods

Take note: 60% of what Americans eat is not food at all. It is ultra-processed food-like substances. This category has made many rich while sentencing generations of humans to illness, debilitation, and difficult lives of chronic disease.

Ultra-processed foods are industrial formulations made entirely or mostly from substances extracted from foods (oils, fats, sugar, starch, and proteins), derived from food constituents (hydrogenated fats and modified starch), or synthesized in laboratories from food substrates or other organic sources (flavor enhancers, colors, and several food additives used to make the product hyper-palatable). Manufacturing techniques include extrusion, molding, and preprocessing by frying. Most beverages may be ultra-processed. Group 1 foods are a small proportion of, or are even absent from, ultra-processed products.[160]

Do *not* trust processed foods to get the chemistry you need. Much of the chemistry we need has been removed, never was there, or worse, toxic chemistries have been deliberately added. Getting enough of the chemistry our biology needs (largely plant and protein) is REALLY important, but arguably more important is eliminating the toxic chemistry from industrial foods from our diets. Look at the ingredient list on a package. How many ingredients are listed? Can you pronounce each word listed? Do you recognize each ingredient as a food you could grow or buy? Remove the poisons of Groups 3 and 4 from your world. Embrace the real, whole foods found in Groups 1 and 2.

Generations of Americans have been conditioned, dare I say manipulated, into eating this toxic waste. Saturday morning cereal cartoons, the 1980s "kid meals," diet foods—all highly processed, all ultimately deadly.[161] As I sit here writing, someone I love is in a hospital fighting for life. Born in the 1980s to a hardworking, low-income single mother, he grew up on frozen pizzas and Pepsi. He had diabetes by age 14 and was on dialysis by age 35. It is a slow, miserable death. It is a painful, miserable life. Obesity, depression, diabetes, heart disease, pain, and cancer all are correlated to ultra-processed food consumption.[162,163] Decades of disease, decades of lost life, decades of misery. Trillions of health dollars spent to treat the impact of ultra-processed food consumption. Until the leaders of our societies have the wisdom and courage to do something about this genocide, *you* must respond. GET MAD! DO NOT EAT PROCESSED FOOD OR ALLOW ANYONE YOU LOVE TO EAT IT!

Reduced Absorption

If you eat a great diet and take a bunch of great supplements, but your gut/body does not absorb them, did you benefit from them? The answer is no. Absorption is the process of getting needed nutrients into the body for use. Anything that interrupts this process can contribute to nutrient deficiency.

As a pharmacist, my job on your health team is about getting results. The physician assesses the problem (diagnoses), and the pharmacists comes up with and monitors the solution. Sometimes that solution involves choosing the best available therapy. Often it involves making (compounding) the best possible therapy, helping with the economics, avoiding bad side effects, offering education and emotional support. The pharmacist must determine the best way to get this therapy into the body, i.e., capsule, intravenous, suppository. The pharmacist's work involves choosing, preparing and monitoring the best therapies to support optimal body function.

Therapies may get into the body through the gut in the dosage form of a capsule, tablet, or a suppository, but sometimes it is through the skin in the form of a cream or injection or IV directly into the bloodstream. In this book, the dosage form we are talking about is food. When thinking of nutrients, it is critical to consider and solve the challenges of getting nutrients absorbed into the body. As we mentioned in the earlier chapters on a healthy and functioning gut, food is THE critical component to getting the needed chemistry into the cellular machines.

Increased Requirements (DEMANDS)

Life and the body are *never* static. Change is the only constant in life. With every heartbeat, you are different. Different challenges, different thoughts, different function. Every day, you must make and spend your body weight in energy (ATP)! Get that 150 pounds of chemistry created and spent EVERY.SINGLE.DAY! How much nutrients/nutrition/energy do you need for life? There are times in life when the body needs more—more sleep, more nutrition, more energy, more grace; there are times when we need less.

Life happens. Life is challenging for all living creatures. Life has a unique way of throwing us curves and demanding more of us. Some call those situations stress. Stress is often thought of as a negative situation. I would like you to consider it is not a negative/positive, good/bad conversation. I like to think of it as what are the "demands" placed on the body. How many "browsers" are up on your computer? The demands on you are very different when on a vacation on the beach for three weeks, compared to being pregnant and giving birth to a human, compared to meeting that last-minute deadline for a boss, compared to navigating a pandemic. Add to that list the demands of taking care of children, unreconciled early-life trauma, all while being severely deficient in the nutritional chemistry to function due to our crazy cultural diet. The result is a computer/body that does not work well; a body that must adjust to merely survive. Increased needs/demands magnify the negative impact of these deficiencies. Beyond "stress," why would the body need more? Infections, pain, toxins, diseases, elections, death of a loved one, the new baby/husband/job, putting on a wedding, change—life is full of times of needing more.

Universal Demands to Begin to Assess

Deficiencies-not enough of something needed (cellular starvation)
Protein, Vitamin D, B-vitamins, Minerals (iron, zinc, magnesium, potassium, sodium), Protein, Omega 3 fats, Hormones, Oxygen, Phytoactive Nutrients, Fiber

Toxicities-too much
Insulin, Sugar, Fructose, Cortisol, Fear

Infections
Virus (Epstein-Barr, Herpes, Covid, Lyme disease, etc.), Fungus (Candida), Mold, Small Intestinal Bacterial Overgrowth (SIBO), Bacterial, Streptococcal, Parasites

Pain
Pain is tremendously demanding on the system, generating severe "fight or flight" stress reactions. Pain is like 10 people yelling at you all of the time. Critical to optimal function is the management and resolution of pain.

It's *critical* to address the root cause. Pain is incredibly demanding on the body.

Sleep

Lack of sleep causes problems; problems cause lack of sleep. Must get to the root cause.

Toxins/Poisons

Often found in doses that do not kill the host but may significantly alter metabolic function.

Alcohol, smoking, pesticides, illicit drugs, medications, environmental pollutants, heavy metals (lead, mercury, arsenic, etc.).

Genetics

Each of us has a unique genetic program that is designed to flex with our environment. In some environments our genetics may be beneficial, in some, not. The modern environment is not conducive to human genetics or health. Because environment (70%) plus genetics (30%) equal physical expression, you have the power to alter your genetic actions with the alteration of your environment (epigenetics).

Exercise/Movement

Too much or too little movement both create challenges for the body.

Psychological

How the brain interprets the world is a powerful determinant of body function. Have you been trained see the world as "half full" or "half empty?" This is an important and modifiable determinant of health and longevity.[164]

Internal Dialog

"No matter what you say to yourself, about yourself, your brain is always listening." If that internal dialog is negative, there may be a negative impact on the physiology; if positive, there may be a positive impact on physiology.[165]

External Dialog

The conversations (press, social media, relationships, etc.) around us influence our brain's perception and subsequent response to stress.

Trauma/Adverse Childhood Events
Trauma alters the physiology until resolved and has tremendous negative impact on health.[166] (See Chapter 19: Famine of Connection.)

As you can tell, that list is just a fraction of the demands that the modern human may face. Recognizing and addressing the demands on your system is a powerful tool in navigating health.

Increased Loss/Use

Imagine a bucket full of water with a small hole. That bucket is essentially our body. There are times that the hole in our bucket—the amount water leaking out—is greater, and times it is smaller. Like those times when you find yourself working out in the yard on a hot day, sweating up a storm. In this case, many of us can recognize the "leaking" of nutrients or electrolytes through our sweat and expended energy with the work we are doing.

The body has an amazing ability to regulate the chemistries of the body—it is a pretty critical function.

There are times when the body increases the excretion or use of chemicals that we may not be as easily aware of. For example, we know that when insulin is high in the body, through administration, or through excessive production in your own pancreas due to a high processed carbohydrate diet, the kidneys will react by getting rid of more potassium and magnesium.[167] You will have an increased loss of critical nutrients secondary to the increased insulin. Low potassium and magnesium may lead to elevations in blood pressure, headaches, arrhythmias, constipation, insomnia, as well as muscle cramping.[168]

Health Strategy

- Identify and manage the "demands" on your system.
- What "browsers" are up on your "computer?" Identify key demands on your system.
- What are you deficient in? Consider getting a laboratory assessment to see in what you may be deficient. Work with your doctor or pharmacist or go to www.ultalabtests/DrKathyHealth.com to order your lab work directly.

Practice

- Take the ACE assessment score[169] Understand that you have survived. Seek out a counselor to understand and resolve traumatic events. You deserve it.
- Optimize your chemistry. Work with a clinical pharmacist and nutritionist to optimize medications and nutrients.
- What have you eaten over the last 24 hours? 7 days? Year? What is your default diet?
- How many cups of "plants" have you consumed in the last 24 hours? 7 days? Listen and log your body's messages.
- What is your body trying to tell you? Do you have:
  - Diarrhea, constipation, bloating, reflux?
  - Fatigue?
  - Headaches?
  - Confusion?
  - Difficulty concentrating?
  - Skin problems?
  - Joint pain?
  - Inflammation?
  - Do you dream? (This could be a clue to how well your body is working during sleep)

CHAPTER 8:

Famine of the Cell

> *"Just one living cell in the human body is more complex than New York City."*
>
> ~Linus Pauling

The medicines you take (or your parents took) could be contributing to your cellular starvation.[170] Unique to the modern human is the daily utilization of modern pharmaceuticals. As a pharmacist, that focus has been much of my life's work. As a pharmacist in one community for over 30 years, I have had the great fortune to have served four generations of patients. I have known many of these patients longer than I knew my own mother! I have watched as many were in decline and as the medications they increasingly took did little to slow the decline, or actually made them worse. That deterioration is when I began to look deeper into and assist my patients with the other chemistries needing to be managed in order to produce health.

Drug-induced nutrient deficiencies occur when the medications we take ***deplete, block absorption, increase excretion,*** or ***increase utilization*** of nutrients resulting in nutrient deficiency. Depletion of critical nutrients can happen as a result of medications being routinely taken. For example, the commonly prescribed cholesterol-reducing class of drugs termed statins reduce the production of the critical energy-producing chemical CoEnzyme Q 10.[171] Through the way we block cholesterol production with statins, we also reduce the production of this nutrient. With the depletion of this nutrient, cellular energy (ATP) production is reduced.

All drugs have unintended and potentially damaging effects. No chemical going into the body is benign. All have some effect, whether intended or unintended. Often, the benefit outweighs the cost, but if you are on medications, it is important that you have a chemistry expert (pharmacist) helping you assess the optimization of ALL of the chemicals going into your body. We need the positive effects from these therapies, but we definitely want a strategy to minimize the damaging effects. Understanding as well as correcting these drug-induced problems is critical. As we noted in Famine of the Gut (Chapter 5), reducing acid in the stomach reduces absorption of nutrients. Acid-blocking medications (proton-pump inhibitors, histamine-2 blockers, anticholinergic medications) have a profound negative effect on the absorption of nutrients from the diet. The immediate "benefit" of, say, reduced acid reflux is seldom fully measured as to the long-term risks of osteoporosis, kidney disease, stroke, dementia, and early death.[172]

As mentioned earlier, increased insulin from a medication or resulting from a high sugar/carbohydrate diet, will increase the excretion/loss of potassium and magnesium through the kidneys.[173] Commonly used diuretics or "water pills" will result in a similar wasting of critical minerals, magnesium, calcium, potassium and sodium. Low levels of these chemicals make it impossible for the body to function without problems. Given that these chemicals are required for muscle contraction, specifically the heartbeat, deficiency in these nutrients can have terrible consequences beyond the commonly experienced muscle cramps, headaches, insomnia and constipation.[174] Survival will require the body to adapt and adjust.

Many medications require more nutrients to process. Estrogen-containing medications (i.e., birth control and hormone replacement), for example, require increased needs for B-vitamins.[175] Taking such medications without accounting for the increased need for nutrients will lead to a deficiency, decreased function, and if left unaddressed, disease.

I am fully aware of the power and benefits of modern pharmaceutical therapies. Without argument, such therapies have been lifesaving for many. But often not discussed or considered are the unintended side effects of their use or overuse. Often, the immediate benefit of a drug is not adequately weighed against the long-term risk.[176] It has been recognized that a major risk factor for developing drug-induced nutrient deficiencies is the lack of awareness by the prescribing physician and a long duration of drug therapy.[177]

Many pharmaceuticals, such as opioids, antibiotics, and anti-inflammatories, have been removed from the market decades after their negative impact of their use is finally recognized.[178] Understanding the true impact of a chemical in the body is a difficult thing as each of us is unique—each situation is unique. What helps or hurts you may not help or hurt me. To have health, you must fully account for the impact that pharmaceuticals are having on your body. I want you not to need medications, but if needed, we must minimize any negative effect that medications may have.

Famine of Care

Do get help to understand and balance the chemistry in your body. Insurance-driven modern health care has, unfortunately, largely removed the chemistry expert, your pharmacist, from your health team. The local pharmacist who knew you and your family is becoming less available. All pharmacists are trained as clinical pharmacists. Many pharmacists have been siloed into big corporate pharmacies, wasting their talents, and creating dangerous barriers between the patient and the pharmacist.[179] Many patients have been forced to receive medications from impersonal corporate pharmacies—or worse, unregulated, dare I say dangerous mail order[180]—never gaining access to the potentially life-saving insights of a pharmacist. Independent or compounding pharmacies often have a clinical pharmacist available for consultation. Seek out a clinical pharmacist to support you. (Like I said, all pharmacists are trained as clinical pharmacists, so don't hesitate to discuss your prescriptions with the staff pharmacist regardless of where you purchase them.) Build that invaluable therapeutic relationship. Your health or your family's may depend on it! (Contact me at www.**drkathysays.com/partner** to find a pharmacist "***Partner in Health***" near you.)

With the modern-day marketing of pharmaceuticals, we have been groomed to believe that the magical medicine from the mailbox is the recipe for health. Nothing can be further from the truth. Health is not taking 15 medications a day; health is much closer to *not needing* 15 medications a day. The evolution of insurance-based, Wall Street-driven health care has resulted in patients' having access to less and less expertise and real care. The current system actually *requires* you to be sick (a diagnosis) in order for any care to be paid for. Yes, disease is subsidized in our society, while health is not. Most of these diagnoses result in a pharmaceutical solution from a system trained to diagnose and treat disease, not prevent need. We are placing more chemicals in our bodies than ever in the history of man, with little or no help from anyone who knows much about chemistry! Cheap drugs cause expensive problems. A relationship with *your* pharmacist can be your greatest weapon in navigating health. Make sure you have one on your team!

Health Strategy

- Optimize your biochemistry!
- Build your health team!
- If you are being prescribed medications from more than one physician, it is very important to consult with your

pharmacist about optimal medication coordination and care.

Practice

- Add to your health timeline the medications you have taken over your lifetime. Also add why you took them.
- Gather all your health information in one place, including recent lab results, lists of medications, and how long you have been taking them and why.
- Write out your health timeline. These clues can help your pharmacist/health team better understand what your body is dealing with.
- Schedule an appointment with a pharmacist today.
- Get a medication/vitamin review today!
- What medications, supplements, chemistries have you taken over the last 10 years?
- Who is your pharmacist?
- Who is helping you with drug-induced nutrient deficiencies?
- When is the last time you spoke with a pharmacist about your medications and their interactions?

CHAPTER 9:

Famine of Fasting

"Fasting is the greatest remedy—the physician within."

~Paracelsus

Periods of "famine," or no food, it turns out, are critical to optimal delivery, processing, and function of the chemistry throughout the cell. The cell has an enormous amount of work to do, and both your life and your health depend on all this work being done.

Consider that cellular assembly line. Food (sugar, fat, protein) comes into the body and is delivered at the cellular loading dock. The cell sends its workers (enzymes, carrier proteins, etc.) to pick up the package and bring it into the cell to be ready for processing. The cellular "workers" begin to process this precious load of nutrients, but the bell on the loading dock rings—another shipment of goods is being delivered to the cell.

The cell stops the processing to bring the additional load into the cell. Soon, the cellular loading dock is packed with goods everywhere. Those stored goods often take the form of stored fat (obesity) or fatty acids as the body's way to handle the incoming until it has time to process.

Because the cell has so much coming in, much of its energy is used to capture and store this precious (and for much of human history, rare) food. The assembly lines to process the goods aren't functioning well to begin with. There's too much being delivered, with no time or workers to process the nutrients into energy. There's no time to "repair" old machines, half the assembly lines are down due to low supply of what the assembly lines actually need to function (nutrients), and there is no time to train new workers.

We modern humans consume or produce sugar continuously. For the cell to actually process this food, we must give it time to process—we must have times of "famine," times of no food. The body has an enormous amount of work to do to keep you alive. Much of this work the body must perform is scheduled over a roughly 24ish-hour clock. This body's daily rhythm, the circadian rhythm, is exquisitely metered throughout the day and night to get this work done. Turns out that food and light conspire to hijack this critical schedule.[181]

Over the last several decades, we have been led to believe we should eat all day to keep our blood sugar stable. That's hogwash. The human body has evolved the ability to go through long periods of time with little or no food. At a minimum, we are designed to go through the night (12 hours) without eating.

Time between meals allows for our cells to really process this food and turn it into the energy needed. During this between-meal fast, the cell works to break down the food and turn the chemicals into energy.

As we occupy our modern life, we find ourselves eating all of the time—coffee with sugar, chips out of the vending machine, candy from the candy bowl, the afternoon pick-me-up, and the bedtime snack.

New research into circadian rhythms has us looking into the age-old customs of fasting. For most of history, fasting, whether nature-driven or through religious traditions, was a routine occurrence for humans. Now, the 24/7 "food" environment of the 20th century, which continues into the 21st century, represents a "dinosaur-ending" environmental shift for humans.

Fasting from food was a daily occurrence as the darkness, directed by sun patterns, naturally dictated our human behaviors. Fasting from food occurred naturally during the months when food availability became less. These times of less nutrition are a time of cellular regeneration,[182] a time when our bodies would identify cells not working well (senescent cells) and recycle (autophagy),[183] a time when our bodies switched into burning stores of fat instead of just burning glucose (metabolic flexibility).[184] Times of little food intake—be it between meals, at night, or during the famine of winter—allowed for normalization of excessive hormones secreted due to previously excessive food and stress. Turns out that this strategy can be valuable for your health too.

Toxic Fructose/Insulin

The research regarding fasting and time-restricted feeding is incredibly exciting. As we work to solve this Modern Famine, we must give our cells the time and the chemistry needed to process the incoming nutrition. At a minimum, an easy first step is to expand your nighttime non-eating period. For some this will be difficult. Most of us have severely elevated levels of the hormone insulin, and suddenly not eating can result in periods of uncomfortable and potentially dangerous low blood sugar.

Survival of the Fattest

Fructose and insulin may be the reason the human species survived. When did primitive man find sugar? As we mentioned earlier, small amounts of glucose are available in green leafy plants. Beyond that, large amounts of sugars are not found very often in nature. With the exception of fighting a bear for honey, you would find sugar primarily toward the end of the annual growing season when fruit would ripen (producing the unique and powerful sugar fructose). Critical to your survival, you (and all animals) would eat as much of it as possible. It is estimated that primates had to gain 50 pounds of fat every fall just to survive the starvation winter![185] If you were lucky, you contained the genetics to produce the chemistry (insulin, fructose, and uric acid) to store that sugar into fat. You would then survive the long winter. You would live to reproduce. We all have the genetics for survival—the genes to get fat.

Fructose, the sugar primarily found in nature as ripened fruit, is a big trigger for the body to begin storing fat for the winter. Rick Johnson, MD, and his team have done tremendous work teasing out what turns out to be the exquisitely elegant biochemical mechanisms of survival.[186] As the growing season progresses through the year, food becomes more plentiful, plants ripen and produce more fructose and carbohydrates. Animals eat more, stimulating an increased use of cellular energy as it processes the incoming fructose/carbohydrates. Fructose initially uses a big chunk of energy (ATP) in order for the cell to process it, compared to the more easily utilized (less energy required) sugar glucose. This decrease/depletion of cellular ATP (energy) results in the production of uric acid, which stimulates fatty acid production (fat storage) as well as hunger, telling the animal (you) to go eat more. Yes, eating fructose actually drives hunger and your wanting more to eat! It's a perfect strategy for surviving the oncoming starvation winter.

Insulin is a *very* powerful hormone. Hormones are basically chemicals with jobs to do. In this case, the key job of insulin is to regulate blood glucose levels. In the pharmacy, insulin is one of the most dangerous, toxic chemicals we dispense.[187] It is also life-giving, but too much insulin can quickly become fatal. Insulin is produced with the ingestion of sugar and will quickly take that sugar out of the bloodstream and into the cell. Too little sugar in the bloodstream or *hypo* (less) *glycemia* (sugar) can quickly occur with too much insulin.[188]

Hypoglycemia is a life-threatening crisis. The brain responds to this low blood sugar crisis by calling a RED ALERT! The heart speeds up, the blood vessels dilate (hot flashes, light headedness, grumpy, anger, rapid heartbeat, irritability). The muscles and liver begin to dump stored sugar into the bloodstream. This drop in blood sugar triggers a "life or death response," and the brain strongly reacts by telling you to GET FOOD NOW OR YOU ARE GOING TO DIE! The brain often "suggests" that you get food immediately. Those strong sugar cravings likely mean that insulin is the issue.

Much like thirst is the body's search for water, a sugar craving is often the body needing something, often it is a search for sugar to neutralize excessive insulin. Even though you have that craving, the brain does not trust you (or the environment) to provide the sugar it needs. It will immediately begin to pump out the stored sugar from the body into the bloodstream.

With low blood sugar, elevated insulin, or times of stress, you will survive by making sugar from the liver.[189] *Gluco* (sugar) *neo* (new) *genesis* (make) is the making of new sugar by the body. With elevated insulin, the body will store sugar made from the liver into fat. You can gain weight without the benefit of eating!

When I think of the power that insulin can have, I think of J., who came to me asking for help. I'd known J. as a patient for decades. We had a good relationship.

She gained 30 pounds eating just 500 measly calories a day and just felt terrible. Many practitioners might be quick to dismiss J. when she said what she was eating, but they'd be wrong to do so. We quickly sat down for an appointment to dig into what might be happening.

J. had been a Type 2 diabetic on large amounts of insulin before she underwent a weight loss surgery 10 years prior. The surgery was very successful, and she was able to discontinue her insulin need and manage her blood sugar with an oral medication called metformin. As we sat down, she told me that six months or so prior, she had a mild heart attack and was taken off of the metformin and put on another oral diabetic medication called glyburide.

Without skepticism, **I believed J.** when she said she had gained 30 pounds eating 500 calories a day. I knew that if she was eating 500 calories a day she was probably only absorbing, at most, 400 calories a day. After all, her weight loss procedure was designed to diminish the nutrition she absorbed. Her body was in crisis! The weight gain was her body's way to survive. Our next step was to figure out why.

In speaking with J., I mentioned the incredible effect that insulin will have on cravings. Most of us think that cravings are conscious, but they are definitely not conscious. Cravings are messages from the starving cell to the primitive brain (the behavior organ) in order to get you to do something (much like how thirst is to get us to drink water). When insulin is high, the wallpaper on the wall begins to look like a tasty treat. Any food and all food will do. The impulse is a deep-brain, unconscious response.

J. nodded. She told me that she slept with a tub of peanut butter by her bed. She would wake from a deep sleep, reach down, grab a spoonful, eat it and go back to sleep. Did she do it because she was lazy and weak? NO! This was the brain keeping her ALIVE! Her primitive brain recognized that her blood sugar was critically low. That response to eat was a survival response.

I suspected that the new drug was the culprit. Glyburide[190] is from a class of diabetic drugs called the sulfonylureas. These are antidiabetic drugs widely used in the management of diabetes mellitus Type 2. They act by increasing insulin release from the beta cells in the pancreas. One of insulin's primary jobs is to drive sugar out of the bloodstream and into the cell.[191]

For J., the new medication increased her insulin production, sending her on a chemical/blood-sugar roller coaster. It was an unregulated, unintended crisis that her body had to adjust to in order to survive. The drug-induced increase in insulin, created low blood sugar crises, thus stimulating her liver to produce sugar (so that she did not die from too little).

This resulted in an increased storage of fat due to the elevated insulin and sugar produced within her system—not related to the 400 calories consumed through her diet.

Sugar Damage

Too much sugar in the bloodstream is a big deal to the body. I remember reading an account from a cardiologist who routinely performed heart bypass surgeries. He commented that when he looks into the blood vessels of a diabetic (someone who routinely has elevated levels of blood sugar in the bloodstream), it looks like someone took a wire brush to the inside of the blood vessel.

There is a process that happens in the body where sugar (glucose, fructose, etc) will chemically bind to a protein, called glycation of proteins, and results in what is termed glycation end products. In the blood vessel, this process will occur when the sugar levels exceed 100 in the blood.

When we measure long-term sugar levels in the blood, we look at the glycation of the red blood cell with a test called the A1C (glycosylated hemoglobin). Interestingly, the sugar fructose binds to proteins 7-10 times more easily than glucose.[192] The A1C test measures the "tail" of sugar connected to the blood cell over the course of its life. The longer the "tail," the higher the circulating levels of sugar in the blood. It may be helpful to think of the sugar glaze on a donut or the sugar coating on a gum drop. An A1C measures how much "glaze" is on the red blood cell.

Consider now that our blood vessels are lined and connected with cells. With an elevated blood sugar, the sugar binds to the "mortar" in between the cells lining the blood vessels. For the body, this binding is very irritating and looks a lot like a scratch. With that "scratch," the body will send in the SWAT team. Just like a scratch on your hand, the body will create swelling and redness inside of the blood vessel. The liver will begin increasing its cholesterol production in order to have the building blocks the irritated tissue needs to repair the sugar's damage to the blood vessel.[193] The immune system will send in cleanup and repair cells to "repair" the scratch.[194] Heart disease is often caused by elevated sugar and this damaging effect on the blood vessels.[195]

Imagine that scratch on the inside of a big, thick blood vessel (think of a fire hose), like the one in your heart. Elevated blood sugar will create many scratches and subsequent repairs inside the vessel. The buildup of cholesterol or plaques in our blood vessels are actually our bodies attempt to repair the damage often caused or at least contributed to by sugar. This damage is the cause of much of our cardiovascular disease. We call this *macro* (big) *vascular* (blood vessel) damage. We know this type of damage is happening years before one is diagnosed with "diabetes."[196]

Now imagine what happens if the blood vessel is one cell thick. Capillaries are the tiniest of blood vessels transporting critical nutrients/oxygen deep into tissues, while at the same time escorting toxins or waste products such as CO_2 (carbon dioxide) out of the tissues.

In this case, I think of a balloon. If the balloon is scratched, it pops or collapses. That damage is exactly what happens to our precious tiny blood vessels (capillaries) when "scratched" by sugar. This is the *micro* (small) *vessel* (blood vessel) damage so prevalent with diabetes and prediabetes. With this sugar damage, we lose the small roads supporting the tissues and cells. The tissues that are highly dependent on these now missing capillaries are subsequently starved and damaged. The resulting disorder is the eye (retinopathy), kidney (nephropathy), and nerve (neuropathy) damage that we are so concerned about in the diabetic patient.[197]

One organ that is hugely affected by this capillary damage, but rarely assessed, is the brain. Some have called Alzheimer's to be Type 3 diabetes for just this reason.[198] It is also why medicine is so focused on reducing sugar levels in the diabetic.

The *big* problem is that the damage has been going on years prior to being diagnosed with sugar issues.[199] Humans are coming out of the womb with too much sugar in our bodies! Our cultural diet is infused with sugar with every bite. Elevated insulin and stress hormones stimulate our livers to make more sugar. We live in a culture that reliably produces blood sugar issues. The body knows such excess is a big deal and tries hard to keep this damage from happening. If you are *lucky*, you have very "thrifty genes" and are very good at producing insulin, getting that sugar out of the bloodstream, and storing these "rare sugar" calories into fat. IF YOU ARE LUCKY, YOU GET FAT! If you are not fortunate to have the genetics of storage, the sugar remains in the bloodstream, causes vascular damage, and you die "thin" of a massive heart attack in your 40s or 50s.

Obesity is the body's attempt to keep going, given the inputs. It is the body's attempt to survive our environment. The human body has not changed—our environment, our culture, has. Too much sugar, too much stress, (another driver of sugar/insulin production), too little nutrients, too little movement are the new norms—the new environment that modern humans are attempting to survive.

While it is key to manage our blood sugar to an optimal range (70-92[200,201]), new research suggests it may be the insulin causing much of the real chaos and, yes, weight gain.[202] In J.'s case, I recommended she and her physician discontinue the unpredictable oral insulin-stimulating medication (glyburide) and begin J. on a small, measurable and adjustable nighttime dose of insulin. The oral medicine could not be controlled as to how low it was driving J.'s blood sugar, especially at night, while the insulin could be more directly monitored and adjusted. Correcting and optimizing her insulin level was the key. The physician and J. agreed to try this strategy. J. came in two weeks later to give me an update and reported "I have my life back."

Assisting patients with diabetes is a big part of what I do as a pharmacist. Because of that need, I have always sought to be as well trained and current in my knowledge of the best strategies. In addition to regular reading of current medical publications, I go to a full weekend training every decade or so, dedicated to learning every new bit of knowledge about diabetes in order to best assist my patients. I will never forget a moment that changed my life forever. Around 2014, I was sitting in that diabetes-focused weekend in Wichita, Kansas, listening to the presenter. She made a comment that rings in my head even today.

"We know diabetes takes 15 years to happen."

REALLY? 15 YEARS?! I thought to myself, "WHY IN THE WORLD DO WE WAIT UNTIL YEAR 16 TO DO ANYTHING ABOUT IT?"

We know that cardiovascular damage is happening 10 years before the diabetes diagnosis![203] We know that the roots of dementia lay within those 15 years. And we (your medical professionals) are doing little to stop this. This situation IS NOT okay by me. I decided I wanted to assist my patients before they became diabetic.

A decade before a diabetes diagnosis, there are clues: weight gain, high blood pressure, inflammation, pain, depression…these symptoms are not just a diagnosis to be medicated—they are critical clues of your body's survival. Many of the "famines" teased out in this book are the modifiable drivers of disease and of the survival of our miraculous bodies.

Critical to this chapter is the concept of less—too much sugar, too much insulin versus times of no sugar, no insulin. We are designed for less, despite living in an environment of "too much of the wrong stuff." If you notice cravings for sugar or carbohydrates and new weight gain, you may be dealing with an elevated insulin issue, driven by early increases in blood glucose. Nevertheless, your blood sugars will be "normal" for years as your body works to survive the insulin/sugar chaos.

Think about when you eat. Begin observing how and what foods your body is asked to process. For some, beginning to introduce periods of no food into their life may be difficult due to the presence of medications or elevated insulin.

We can begin to rebalance our system by not eating between meals, reducing the sugar we consume, and work to reduce the stress-induced sugar production. Alter how you stimulate insulin by limiting your consumption of those foods containing sugar…that soda, candy bar, cereal, or mocha. Once insulin begins to improve, look to expand your nighttime "no eating window." Can you go 6 hours, 8 hours, 10 hours, 12 hours without food at night? Introducing times of "no food" to our body is an exciting and simple way to support our health to create the famine our body actually needs.

Health Strategy

- Add periods of 'no food' to one's day.
- Optimize blood sugar.

Practice

- Audit your daily carbohydrate and sugar intake.
- How much fiber do you consume?
- Calculate the net carbs in what you routinely eat.
- What are your body clues? (Diagnosis?)
- Note on your timeline when you first began to gain weight?
- When do you eat?
- How many hours do you go without eating?
- Do you often snack throughout the day?
- What is your fasting insulin level on your blood work?
- What is your A1C?
- Are you on medications that alter your insulin or sugar

level?
- Consider proactive continuous blood glucose monitoring to understand how your body is processing sugar through the day. (See drkathysays.com/cgm for more information.)

CHAPTER 10:

Famine of Flavor

"Fat gives things flavor."

~Julia Child

If sugar stimulates insulin and insulin stimulates chaos, where does all the sugar come from? Sugar comes from two sources: what we take in through the mouth and what we create in the liver.

Remember, food is chemistry. This chemistry is critical information that directs your body function. We went over earlier how fat became the villain of health and sugar became the savior during the 1980s SnackWell's Revolution.[204] People wanting to make healthy choices sought out low-fat solutions. Unfortunately, manufacturers found that the removal of fat from "foods" led to the removal of flavor and satisfaction. More sugar to the rescue.

Sugar manufacturers could not keep up with their newly created demand via the traditionally grown cane or beet sugar. High-fructose corn sweetener was created in the 1970s[205] and became a cheap way to fuel the new need for flavor. What humans consider food changed forever and fueled the profound shift in what humans eat and in human health.

Also created to deal with this new flavor dilemma was the no-calorie sweetener industry. The early 1980s brought the explosion of diet sodas.

Marketed as "safe and healthy," no one at the time knew what the long-term impacts would be. We are just now, 40 years later, beginning to comprehend the damaging shift that these foreign chemicals have had on the human body.[206]

Contrary to what you might believe from advertisements, it is **not** good to consume products with diet or artificial sweeteners in them. It's better to stick with moderate amounts of the sweeteners nature made, like the unprocessed sugars found in whole fruit and honey.

The consequences of these "diet chemicals" have been tragic. Those consequences have impacted me personally—and it makes me very angry.

As I said, at five years old, I weighed 100 pounds. Other than water, I was only allowed to drink diet soda. I was a TAB girl, then Diet Coke, then Diet Dr. Pepper. For 45 years they were my preferred beverages—until I began to read the research suggesting those diet sodas may have contributed to my weight struggles.[207] Non-nutritive sweeteners or "diet" sugars have been implicated in contributing to obesity by altering the metabolism, disrupting the microbiome, and stimulating the brain's craving of sweetened foods.[208] In good faith, I was making a best effort to be healthy by avoiding "real" soda and choosing diet. The truth is that both are toxic and can make you fat.[209]

Health Strategy

- Eat REAL, flavorful food.

Practice

- Food should taste great! It does not have to be bland or boring to be good for you. You can and should enjoy the foods you eat.
- Spices and herbs add great flavor (and medicinal

chemistries) to the foods you eat. If you love garlic, consider adding garlic to your meal. While you are at it, give basil, parsley, lemon, tumeric, black pepper, and so much more, a try. (Check out my line of salts and spices developed to make this easier! **store.drkathysays.com**)

- Acids such as lemon juice and vinegars can bring great flavor to many dishes.
- Do not be afraid to include high-quality, delicious fats in your diet. Avocado, nuts, olives, fatty fish are delicious and nutritious. Make sure your diet contains some of these every day.
- List what 10 things do you buy and eat all of the time.
- Specify how you season your foods.
- Note from what sources you get sugar.
- Track how often do you buy and eat heat-and-serve food instead of cooking raw products.
- Take note of artificial flavorings and additives and eliminate them whenever possible.

CHAPTER 11:

Famine of Fiber

"Think of fiber as 'nature's broom' for the body."

~Unknown

As a mom of two girls, I was blessed to have been exposed to a decade of Disney movies. One of my favorites is *Finding Nemo*. In one scene, Nemo finds himself with fellow "prisoners" in a fish tank, plotting their escape. Their strategy included getting out and heading for the sink drain, as "All drains lead to the ocean."

With regard to what we eat, **all carbohydrates lead to sugar.**[210]

Carbohydrates are not in themselves bad and actually are necessary for health. They are basically complex sugars—many single sugar molecules linked together or linked together with other chemical components. Plants provide carbohydrates. Plants also provide us large amounts of the chemicals needed to process the carbohydrates toward energy (ATP) production, B-vitamins, minerals, phytonutrients, etc. When we eat refined/processed carbohydrates—sugar—we are basically eating the sugar with the other needed stuff removed!

With a diet of processed food, we lose fiber. Fiber consists of the parts of plants that your body cannot digest. Fiber is critical because it makes food pass quickly through your body and regulates the absorption of sugar into the body. Fiber impacts how much sugar enters the bloodstream. No fiber, lots of sugar. High fiber, low sugar. THIS IS A BIG DEAL.

Fibers are generally categorized as being soluble or insoluble. Soluble fibers are fibers that can dissolve, are recognized for their ability to lower LDL ("bad") cholesterol, and help control blood sugar. Fruits, legumes, and oats (**PLANTS**) are rich sources of soluble fibers. Insoluble fibers, like those found in wheat, bran, vegetables, and fruits (**PLANTS**) are fibers that do not dissolve and have been linked to health benefits such as appetite control, reduced incidence of developing Type 2 diabetes, and the prevention of constipation.[211]

Another important role of fiber is its ability to act as prebiotics—substances that alter the types and activities of the bacteria, or microflora, that live inside the human gut. Basically, fiber feeds the gut bacteria. Remember, a well-functioning gut microbiome acts as a vitamin factory for your body. The fiber that you cannot absorb is the fiber that feeds the bacteria that makes your vitamins. Happy and well-fed bacteria help make for a healthy host (human).

The human gut bacterial universe remains an exciting area of scientific research. The relationships of this microbial universe to inflammation, immune function, and body health are promising areas for understanding how fiber may offer protective effects against a variety of diseases.[212]

Sugar or carbohydrates should come into the body in the form of plants. Many suggest that diets take in low or no sugar or carbohydrates. In the management of elevated blood sugars, a low carbohydrate approach can be very therapeutic and beneficial in actually reversing the disease.[213] Many popular low-carb diets *do* remove much of the processed foods and sugars from our diet, which is great. But unfortunately, these approaches often remove much of the fiber and micronutrients present in plants necessary for proper cellular and microbiome function. The fiber, carbohydrates, and micronutrients from plants provide us the critical chemicals that our assembly lines and our bacterial friends need to work. In my decades studying "what to eat," I found curious the research that suggested humans lived longer on diets that include beans and whole grains.[214] Those are carbohydrates! How can carbs be healthy? We do not need to eat sugar to live, but we critically need the other fibrous parts of plants from where sugar naturally comes, such as the is the case with beans and whole grains.

The Basics

As early humans evolved, survival often depended on the body's ability to be very flexible and very thrifty. During times of great food, it would store precious nutrients for later, and in times of little food, it could temporarily make do. It turns out this metabolic flexibility is an exciting new way to view health and disease.[215]

Gluconeogenesis (*sugar-new-make*) is the body's making of sugar from non-sugar foods. When little food is available, the body can recycle stored fat and protein components and make sugar newly in the liver. That ability was really important when food was scarce or during times of threat (fight or flight). The body is stimulated to make new sugar by the hormones glucagon, HGH (human growth hormone), epinephrine, and cortisol.

The sugar-generating regulator is where the chaos gets crazy. If you have elevated epinephrine (also called adrenalin), or elevated cortisol often present during times of stress or threat, your body will make sugar. Elevations in blood sugar will trigger insulin production. With elevated insulin levels, your body is directed to remove the damaging levels of sugar out of the bloodstream and store it into fat.

When those hormones are elevated, regardless of what you eat, you will store fat, gain weight, and often feel like junk. Yes, stress can make you fat! Add to this situation our cultural eating of processed food with little fiber and few nutrients. The combination results in large amounts of sugar within the bloodstream, cellular starvation, thus increasing this fat-storage and chemistry chaos. Not eating (fasting or time restricted eating) helps to break this vicious cycle. Not eating the same thing all the time helps too. Eating large amounts of fiber-rich plants helps to slow the sugar dump into the bloodstream. As you audit your unique situation throughout this book, you will see small areas that you can adjust that will make huge health improvements and get out of this vicious cycle.

Health Strategy

- Follow a plant-focused, high-fiber approach.

Practice

- Most people don't get enough fiber. On average, Americans only get about 16 grams of fiber per day. For women, 25 grams per day is recommended, with 38 grams per day recommended for men. [216] Shoot for 10gm per meal or at least 25 grams per day.
- Take a carb and fiber audit.
- Read/study nutrition labels.

Do you know how much fiber you're getting each day? Start keeping track!

To get a sense of what kind of impact fiber has on your system, take how many grams of carbohydrates you ate in the last 24 hours (or at your last meal) and subtract the number of grams of fiber you consumed in the same time period. Total carbohydrates minus fiber equals net carb consumption. The net carb consumption is roughly how many carbohydrates your body absorbs.

How do you feel after a low fiber meal? After a higher fiber meal? Note these things in your health journal. For those monitoring their blood glucose, what is the impact of fiber/lack of fiber on your blood glucose levels?

Begin to consider the role that stress may be contributing to your health/weight.

CHAPTER 12:
Famine of Water

"Water is the driving force of all nature."
~Leonardo da Vinci

Food is the chemistry of life, and water is the soup that makes that the chemistry work. It appears life began in water, and life's existence is absolutely dependent on the presence of that water. For all living things, having a clean reliable source of water is a daily priority. The human body is over 60% water! No water, no life. Wars have been fought and people have died over access to this precious resource. Why is it so important, and how have we messed up this valuable resource so badly?

As a pharmacist, I had to attend and ***pass*** many, many, many chemistry courses. Understanding how a medication works in the body first begins with a strong foundation as to how chemistry works in the world. When thinking of chemical molecules, think of a magnet. We all have played with magnets, noticed the push (positive charge or protons) or the pull (negative charge or electrons) that they make. Each chemical molecule has a unique charge, a unique ability to push or pull—a unique energy. Energy is the ability to move stuff, primarily electrons. Like a wonderful dance couple, this movement seems like magic. With chemistry, we quickly forget the complexity or "magic" and begin to use that magnetic force just to put that picture on the refrigerator or to move that heavy object.

Water is uniquely wonderful, as it contains both the "push force" and the "pull force." Water, good old H_2O, is made up of a negatively charged oxygen molecule (puller) and two weakly positive hydrogen molecules (pushers).[217] Together they *almost* completely neutralize each other.

"Almost" here means that hydrogen is always looking for another dance partner. The weak push or bond of hydrogen is arguably the key to life! While hydrogens like their dance partner (oxygen), they are fickle and will very easily jump around and dance with other chemicals. In addition to oxygen, hydrogens really like nitrogen, sulfur, and other hydrogens.

Oxygen, on the other hand, is very attractive (pull) and has a particular preference for carbon. It is through these "magnetic, push-pull forces" that chemicals come together to make compounds, which come together to make cells, which ultimately come together to make you. Our energy currency—ATP—that we spoke of earlier requires a remarkable 13 molecules of oxygen per molecule of ATP! NO OXYGEN, NO ATP, NO LIFE! Oxygen, water (dihydrogen oxygen), and carbon dioxide (CO_2) represent this dance of life. The unique chemical qualities and presence of water is foundational to life—foundational to you!

Dilution Is the Solution to Pollution

Have you ever tried to dissolve a cup of sugar with a teaspoon of water? It does not work very well. If you don't have enough water to dissolve the sugar, it can mess up the whole chemistry experiment.

Consider salt, for instance. Medicine attributes a lot of body damage to salt (sodium chloride), but often salt alone isn't the true culprit. Actually, the chemicals that make up table salt—sodium and chloride—are critical to body function and essential to life.[218] Salt and the amounts of salt in the body are masterfully utilized and controlled in the body, primarily through the kidney. It turns out that salt without enough water is the big problem.

Imagine drinking a tablespoon of salt in an ounce of water. Yuck! Besides being disgusting, it would burn. Now imagine that same tablespoon of salt in a gallon of water. It would taste fine.

When we eat large amounts of salt with very little water, like we do with the modern Western processed food diet, there is an increased concentration (osmolality) of salt in our bloodstream. That outcome causes our body to react to the "burn," resulting in elevated blood pressure and over time even the production of fructose. Yes, high salt concentrations will cause our body to make sugar! Over time, that effect can cause many problems, one of them being an increase in body weight.[219]

Each cell depends on having enough water in it to have your chemicals dance. These unique electron forces run our chemical assembly lines. It does not hurt that water lubricates the joints and eyes, aids digestion, flushes out waste and toxins, and keeps the skin healthy. Or that water contains some of that critical nutrient called oxygen! YOU NEED WATER—clean water for all bodily functions!

What Is Clean Water?

Humans have been building their lives around clean sources of water for thousands of years. Traditionally, humans have consumed water from the sky or the ground. "Clean sources of water" refer to water without contaminants. Sources of water contamination include naturally occurring chemicals and minerals (arsenic, radon, uranium), local land use practices (fertilizers, pesticides, concentrated feeding operations), manufacturing processes (plastics, fluoride, chlorine), sewer overflows, or wastewater releases.[220]

We all are affected by water contamination. We only have to look to Flint, Michigan to learn that drinking water can be contaminated at the source but also from the distribution system. Old lead-based plumbing introduced the strong "chemical magnet" of lead in Flint's water supply, leaving some residents, including young, developing children, with severe neurological damage.[221] Infants, young children, pregnant women, the elderly, and people whose immune systems are compromised because of AIDS, chemotherapy, or transplant medications may be especially susceptible to illness from contaminants, but consumption of contaminated water impacts us all.

Bottled water isn't much better.

The bottling of water is not particularly new. The 1700s saw the beginning of bottling water and the sale of "artesian" waters with special properties. Large water cooler bottles have been popular for most of the 20th century. The 1980s brought the beginning of a remarkable commercial shift to the individually packaged bottle of water.

The commoditization/marketing of this natural resource has had some unintended consequences to our health. One, it has made water more expensive. "Why should we pay for water when we can pay for something more 'valuable' like a soda or a latte?" That notion has been a subtle change in our thoughts, habits, and preferences on drinking water. We just do not like it as well. Our taste palette, newly trained to the sweet drinks of the 20th century, just does not like water. We also now question the quality of the water coming out of our tap. Generations have now been born, who unlike their grandparents, do not think to drink water from the well, stream, garden hose, or even faucet.[222] It's believed that tens of millions of Americans today don't typically drink water from the tap.[223]

No Famine of Plastics

Another, bigger issue with the bottled water movement are the plastic chemicals used to package bottled water and the impact they have on your body. The creation and utilization of the plastic bottles has a significant environmental impact. Just making the bottle can introduce chemicals into our environment and potentially into our bodies with damaging effects.

More concerning than the environmental impact is the impact of the plastics on the body itself. Whenever you drink out of a plastic bottle, or cook in plastic, you risk ingesting the chemicals used to make the bottles. That danger is particularly common with older plastic water bottles and/or those that have been exposed to heat. BPA and other plastic toxins can then make their way into your bloodstream. BPA stands for bisphenol A, which is an industrial chemical that has been used to make certain plastics and resins since the 1960s. BPAs mimics estrogen and are disruptors to normal hormonal function.[224] Because of this hormone disruption, we are seeing infertility in both men and women, as well as negative impacts on developing children.[225]

Water bottles containing BPA have also been linked to increased rates of disease in adults.[226] Humans with the highest concentrations of BPA in their urine are three times more likely to suffer from cardiovascular disease and 2.4 times more likely to have Type 2 diabetes than are people with low BPA concentrations.

More importantly, and the main reason you are reading this book, is the fact that these plastics have been linked to obesity. Yes, your obesity may be due at least in part to the plastics you have ingested over your life. Hormones are chemicals produced in the body with jobs to do. Estrogen's job is to grow something—hips, breasts, or follicles (eggs) BABY! It is also very helpful to the body (for men and women) to help grow brain, bone, and cardiovascular tissues. All important stuff!

Because these plastics, BPA and others, look and act like estrogen, they can go into the body and mess things up. They are major hormone disrupters. These compounds have been tied to weight-management problems in men and women. Exposure to the compounds in plastic water bottles can ultimately influence the rate at which and where fat is stored in your body and will look a lot like weight gain or difficulty losing weight.

One animal study looking at weight and toxins (in this case persistent organic pollutants, or POPs) remarkably found that the animal seemed to build fat to store the toxins in order to apparently reduce their negative impact on critical cells and tissues, limiting their systemic toxicity.[227] The body in all of its wisdom may increase fat to protect you from these damaging toxins.

As stated earlier, the body does exactly what is necessary to survive. Could the obesity epidemic—your weight gain—be related to plastics and the massive introduction into our bodies of toxic, disruptive chemicals? Yes. That link is becoming clearer and clearer.[228] Plastics and many of the modern chemicals that humans now routinely ingest have created unimaginable biochemical chaos.

Obesity is the symptom.

Health Strategy

- De-toxify your life.

Practice

- Look at the various sources of contaminants in your life, your home, and your food preparation.
- Remove the plastics from your life!
- Never cook or heat food in plastic containers. Switch to glass or ceramic containers for food storage. I love using and reusing Mason jars.
- Evaluate your cookware. Eliminate "non-stick Teflon coated" or aluminum cookware. Consider using quality stainless steel, glass, or cast iron for less-toxic cooking.
- Avoid drinks that are bottled and stored in plastic.
- Avoid or limit the use of scented products.
- Consider a carbon-based filtration device for drinking water.

- Make sure you are eliminating well (pee, poop, sweat, breathing) in order to assist the body's removal of potentially harmful toxins. Clear urine is a good indicator of toxin removal. Remember, the main ways that things leave the body is to pee, poop, sweat or breathe. Make sure you are doing all VERY WELL!
- Increase your vegetable content to 7-10 cups of non-starchy vegetables daily in order to assure enough fiber to help remove toxins and reduce their damaging impact.[229]
- Drink contaminant-free, filtered water (60-100 ounces per day).

Dehydration

As I mentioned earlier, the body is a lot like a bucket with a hole in the bottom, and dehydration happens when your body uses or leaks out more water than you take in. When the normal water content of your body is reduced, it upsets the balance of minerals (salts and sugar) in your body, which totally messes up the way the body functions.

We need just the right amount of water. We can't have too much, and we will not live long with too little. I call this a Goldilocks situation. How much is the perfect amount? Well, it depends.

Think about the bucket. If you have a big hole in the bottom, you will need more water going in to keep your bucket full. Let's assume at this point that you like water, have access to, and will drink plenty of clean, non-contaminated water. How much water you will need will be influenced by how much you use—how much is leaking out of your bucket. The human body will lose water during breathing or in the form of sweat, tears, vomiting, urine, or diarrhea.

Just living our Western sedentary life, we lose about two cups of water a day in sweat, one cup a day through breathing, and about six cups a day in urine.

When you don't get enough water, or lose too much water, you become dehydrated. If your urine is bright yellow, you might not be drinking enough water. Signs of mild dehydration include dry mouth, excessive thirst, dizziness, lightheadedness, and weakness. If people don't get fluids at this point, they can experience severe dehydration, which can cause convulsions, rapid breathing, a weak pulse, loose skin, and sunken eyes. Ultimately, dehydration can lead to heart failure and death.[230]

We can get about 20% of our need for water through whole food but require approximately eight cups of water a day just to get close to replacing that which we use. Anything that increases the "hole in the bucket" (your loss of water) will increase your need to take in more water or make more severe the impact of not enough water. Exercise, manual labor, heat, illness, and medications will cause your body to use more water and make it more important than ever to drink it.

Sneaky Ways You Are Losing Water

It may be obvious that when we exercise or are in a hot environment we sweat more and will need more water. Modern culture has challenged our bodies in new ways that make our dehydration much worse and in ways that may not be so obvious. The increased sugar in our bloodstream since the 1970s has created quite the burden for the body. As we mentioned earlier, high concentrations of sugar are directly damaging to the blood vessel. The body knows it must get rid of this toxic sugar. In addition to pumping out a big dose of insulin, the body will increase the hole into the bucket in order to get rid of this toxin. The kidneys will stop re-absorbing water and send extra water and sugar (and critical electrolytes) out of the body.[231]

The body is amazing and always doing exactly what it deems necessary to survive. If the body is lacking adequate water, it will work to make its own. It will store fat to break it down to water later. Just being dehydrated could be a cause in your holding onto weight!

Modern Drinks

Somewhere over the last 50 years, drinking water has seemingly become optional or strangely, alternative. Nothing is new about humans working to make water more enjoyable or even safer. There have been times in history where drinking fermented beer or wine was safer than drinking potentially contaminated water! For over 5,000 years, the Chinese have been boiling their water with plants, teas, and herbs in order to improve flavor, decrease bacteria, and extract the wonderful and often medicinal chemistry of the plant. Beyond the obvious caffeine in tea or coffee, the hundreds of chemicals pulled from plants during boiling are complex and often complementary to our body's function.

The 20th century might be called the "Century of Soda." From the development of the glass bottle, to the aluminum can, to the plastic container, to the pharmacist-created special syrups (Dr. Pepper and Coca-Cola), to the no-calorie diet drinks, to the dyed drink, the 1900s fundamentally changed what humans think to drink.[232]

What began as an occasional treat, maybe a 12-ounce bottle once a month, or at most once a week, was often more like 32 to 64 ounces a day by the year 2000! While the amount of soda consumed has diminished slightly during the 2010s, Americans are still drinking far too much of it.

Consider the recommendation that we consume in total no more than 30 grams of added sugar daily, which is roughly six teaspoons of sugar.[233] One 12-ounce can of sweetened soda has 40 grams or eight teaspoons of sugar! That is just one can!

Then the 1980s brought the introduction of caffeine into soft drinks. Whether in coffee, tea, energy drinks, or soda, we like our caffeine. It is the world's most widely used psycho- (brain) active drug, and it is legal and unregulated in most parts of the world. Make no mistake: Caffeine is a drug with addictive tendencies. It is a central nervous system stimulant that reduces fatigue and drowsiness. At normal doses, caffeine has effects on learning and memory and generally improves reaction time, wakefulness, concentration, and motor coordination. Caffeine is a drug with which humans have self-medicated for thousands of years.

In addition to caffeine's effects on the brain, caffeine is a diuretic to the body.[234] A diuretic is a drug that stimulates the kidney to rid the body of fluid. Diuretics promote the removal from the body of water, salts, poisons, and accumulated metabolic products, such as urea. A diuretic can alter the fluid balance in the body, resulting in dehydration. Our society's shift away from drinking water and toward caffeinated drinks has left us increasingly dehydrated.

It is not your imagination that it is hard to stop consuming sugar-laden drinks, as well as those with caffeine. Manufacturers have carefully crafted products that leave you dehydrated, tired, hungry, and wanting more. Intense sweeteners, high-fructose corn syrups, plus added caffeine create the experience to be intensely pleasurable, highly addictive, and incredibly dangerous. Best-case scenario for sugar-sweetened drinks is that they will "only" cause obesity. Worst case is metabolic disease, insulin resistance, non-alcoholic fatty liver disease, and early death.[235]

Just one to two sweet drinks a day could be *deadly*. And for the record, diet sodas are not much better.[236]

Just in case you are not convinced to drink water, consider that the fat your body is storing is so the body will always have a source of water. Yes, the body can and will use fat in order to be broken down into metabolic water! Drink water so that your body does not store fat!

Health Strategy

- HYDRATE! Drink Water!

Practice

- Know the symptoms of dehydration.
- Do you:
  - Feel thirsty and lightheaded?
  - Have a dry mouth?
  - Feel tired?
  - Have bright yellow, dark(er) yellow, brown urine?
- Record what you drank in the last 24 hours
- How much caffeine have you consumed?
- How much sugar in all forms have you ingested?
- What types of containers do you use? Small/large bottles? Plastic? Metal? Glass?
- LIMIT SWEETENED DRINKS TO LESS THAN ONE PER MONTH!
- Do not let others sweeten your drinks. Incorporate green tea or other unsweetened herbal drinks instead.
- Aim to drink the equivalent of half of your body weight in ounces of water, up to 100 ounces a day.
- Need flavor in your water? Add vegetables such as cucumbers or fruit such as lemons, limes, oranges, or berries to filtered water for a delicious treat.

Using a tape measure, measure your waist and measure your hips. These numbers (waist to hip ratio) can suggest you may have metabolic dysfunction. If your waist is larger than your hips, STOP all refined sugar immediately.

CHAPTER 13:

Famine of Oxygen

*"Oxygen is **the** essential nutrient."*

~Kathy Campbell, PharmD

Oxygen is critical for the existence of most life. Oh, how we take for granted that deep breath of air and all that it provides. Nothing freaks the body out like not having enough oxygen! Fundamental to ATP production as well as cellular respiration, oxygen is the chemical that fuels our life.

Oxygen is required to keep a fire going—remove the oxygen, and the fire can't survive. It is within your cellular factories, the mitochondria where the presence of oxygen flames your ATP fire.

The journey of oxygen from that deep breath all the way to your mitochondria is long and chemically complex. Breakdowns, or hiccups at any point in this journey, will result in health challenges, and, yes, obesity.[237] We breathe to bring oxygen into our cells and remove waste products (carbon dioxide) from our bodies. Nutrient deficiencies, not having enough of the chemistry needed to transport and use oxygen, is an under-recognized contributor to obesity.

Again, consider iron, for example. Iron is important for normal growth development and function. One important way your body uses iron is to create hemoglobin, a protein in your red blood cells that uses four iron molecules to receive the oxygen you breathe in and deliver it throughout your body and to cellular assembly lines for ATP production. Underappreciated is the role of iron as a critical component on that ATP assembly line. Yes, it is important to have enough iron to make red blood cells, but it is equally as important to have enough iron to make ATP.[238]

Yet, iron deficiency is one of the most common nutrient deficiencies in the world.[239] Often, such deficiency is mild enough that it goes unnoticed for quite some time. Latent iron deficiency can occur for years before the body is no longer able to make adequate hemoglobin, leading to the more readily diagnosed iron deficiency anemia.[240] Symptoms typically include fatigue, chest pain, shortness of breath, cold hands and feet, brittle nails, strange cravings (like for ice), and more.

Doctors are often quick to check for iron with the obvious culprits, such as blood loss from an injury or heavy menstruation. Pregnancy is also a common cause of deficiency. Often, however, low iron or low nutrients in general are missed or never considered as a contributor to your fatigue, depression, or obesity.

Your diet, genetics, and gut health play huge roles in how much iron/nutrients you maintain. Many of us get our iron from red meat, but it can also come from seafood, dark leafy greens, beans, dried fruit, and more.

What if you're eating all that to no avail?

Some people have trouble absorbing iron. Usually, it's absorbed into the bloodstream by way of the small intestine. But if your gut is challenged as in the case with celiac disease or if part of your small intestine has been removed or bypassed for some reason, you might have a harder time absorbing the stuff that keeps you moving. Some of us genetically may absorb too much or too little iron, as in the case of hemochromatosis, each creating its own set of challenges. If you think you may be having unrecognized issues with iron, check with your doctor to get a laboratory assessment with a complete iron panel (including ferritin) before you chose to try to address it yourself. ***Remember, the only thing worse than too little iron is too much iron!***

Iron is just *one* of the critical nutrients that cells require to use oxygen, make energy, and function well. The best strategy is to eat and absorb large amounts of nutrient-dense foods. You can give your body a boost by consuming foods that contain Vitamin C (acid) when you eat iron-rich foods. Thanks to beautiful chemistry at work, Vitamin C helps transform that iron rock so that your body can better absorb it.

Tomatoes, lemon juice, peppers, broccoli, and grapefruit all are foods high in Vitamin C.[241] Combine these foods with iron-rich foods: spinach, beef, eggs, and lentils to make a delicious and nutritious iron solution.

Famine of Clean Air

What about the air itself? The air we breathe is largely composed of different gasses, with oxygen making up a relatively smaller portion at 21%.[242]

According to the Centers for Disease Control and Prevention, particulate matter air pollution is a big deal. It's associated with diminishing lung function, worsening asthma, and increasing premature deaths.[243] Poor air quality or air pollution has a very negative effect on your body in terms of receiving the oxygen critical to health.

Assuming that nothing major changes with government regulations or the general population, the CDC estimates there will be 1,000 to 4,300 additional premature deaths annually by 2050 due to health effects caused by air pollution.[244, 245]

Beyond those numbers, the National Institute of Environmental Health Sciences has found that air pollution impacts everything from obesity, to diabetes, to cardiovascular disease, to immune system disorders, Alzheimer's dementia, and more.[246] We'd be wise to begin to consider the quality of the air we breathe and its impact on our health. The air that you breathe within your home or work place can be improved with HEPA filtration.

Health Strategy

- Increase your cellular oxygen.

Practice

- BREATH! We can no longer take oxygen for granted if we want to be well.
- Reduce toxins in your environment.
- Use HEPA filtration filters in heating and cooling systems.
- Limit or avoid "scented" products (candles, fabric softeners, etc.) from use.
- Evaluate your micronutrient status (iron, B-vitamins, etc.) with a laboratory assessment.
- Get evaluated for sleep apnea if you snore (reduced nighttime oxygenation).
- BREATHE!

You might also consider trying out some meditative breathing exercises, incorporating some gentle yoga into your routine, or even practice singing to increase your lung capacity!

Consider trying diaphragmatic breathing,[247] also known as belly breathing. While this breathing technique can be especially helpful if you have COPD, it's an exercise that can help all of us breathe deeply. Start by relaxing your shoulders while sitting back or laying down. Put one hand on your stomach and one on your chest. Inhale deeply through your nose for a couple of seconds, feeling your stomach expand. Your stomach should move more than your chest. Breathe out, again through your nose, for a couple seconds. Repeat.[248]

You can also develop your lungs by playing a wind instrument or by singing.

CHAPTER 14:

Famine of Movement

"Nothing happens until something moves."

~Albert Einstein

I hate exercise and rarely recommend exercise for my patients. Let me explain. Exercise is an emotional weapon used in our society (and modern medicine) to praise those who do it and shame those who don't. It is also a multibillion-dollar industry.[249] Human beings did not evolve "exercising," just as humans were never designed to sit at a desk or in front a screen for 8-14 hours a day. Based on research of the last primitive peoples on our planet, the estimate is that our ancestors hunted and gathered at a moderate to vigorous pace 6+ hours a day.[250] Exercise is a relatively modern concept created to compensate for the fact we no longer have to use our bodies to live. Believe it or not, the people who live the longest around the globe do not "exercise." They do, however, move.

In his book, *The Blue Zones*, Dan Buettner wrote on his groundbreaking research looking to find the cultures around the world that produce the greatest population of centenarians. Within the cultures, key lifestyle similarities emerged, one of which was that none of these centenarians exercised. They did, however, live lives that "nudged them into movement" every 20 minutes. They move.[251]

Remember from the Famine of Chemistry (Chapter 7), oxygen is critical to energy production. Once oxygen is picked up at the lung by the iron-rich red blood cell, it begins the journey through the bloodstream to the tissues to ultimately be deposited into the cell. The heart is a muscular pump propelling oxygen-rich blood toward the cell and oxygen-depleted blood back toward the lungs to pick up a new load of oxygen. It goes without saying that the heart is critical to life and the circulation of oxygen, but what many may not realize is that the heart is not the only muscle that propels oxygen around the body. All muscles pump blood! With each heartbeat and each movement, blood fills and stretches elastic blood vessels, and blood is circulated. With every movement we make, we are escorting oxygen in and waste products out. If only the heart is available for oxygen circulation, as is the case with the modern sedentary human, lower levels of oxygen may result at the cell, leading to diminished energy production (slowed metabolism). The heart alone was never designed to be the only muscle that pumped blood.[252] We were designed to move.

People often think you have to exercise for all different reasons, ranging from looking good in a bikini, to needing to run a marathon, to reaching some sort of predetermined step count to be "healthy." But I think we're missing a big piece of the puzzle. The reality is that we need to move to propel oxygen (and other nutrients) through the body, deeper into every tissue, deeper into the brain, deeper into each and every cell. If we don't move our bodies, the heart is often overly tasked with doing all that work, and frankly it is not designed to do this important task alone.

We need to move to have a body that works. Below are four types of movements that should be understood and factored into your daily health strategies.

Balance and Stability

Balance is basically your brain connecting you to the ground. The coordination of the nervous system and the musculoskeletal system resulting in balance represents one of the many incredibly intricate, exquisite, and incredibly important biological systems for living a long life. We begin to lose our balance in our 40s. One in three adults over the age of 65 will experience a fall, often leading to debilitating pain and/or hastening illness or death. Balance issues can be a result of blood pressure issues, neurological decline with slowing of reflexes, loss of muscle mass, or medication use.[253] A sedentary life, one where sitting makes up most of the day, has the brain "practice" balance less often. Movement of any kind will stimulate the brain and reinforce balance. Walking, yoga, tai chi, and dancing all are great at maintaining and training your balance muscle. If you already notice challenges with your balance, check with your physical therapist/health team member for specific balance-promoting strategies.

Health Strategy

- Build balance.
- Include a physical therapist on your health team to assist in improving your movement and balance.

Practice

- Try this simple test next to a chair or a wall to evaluate balance:
  - Stand up and imagine you're going to walk forward in a straight line, placing one foot directly in front of the other so that the heel of your front foot touches the toes of your back foot.

> - Keep both feet flat on the floor. Hold that position, and close your eyes.
> - If you can maintain your balance for 30 seconds, you are doing pretty well. If you are wobbling just about as soon as you close your eyes—or before—your balance is poor.
> - Stand on one foot as you brush your teeth in the morning or at other convenient times.
> - Stand back next to a wall, lift your toes, and lean on your heels.
> - Incorporate dance, tai chi, and/or yoga into your day.

Tote and Fetch

We must lift heavy stuff!! "Tote and fetch" represents muscle-building resistance training. Our ancestors lifted heavy things all day every day—babies, game, wood, food—anything necessary for them and their offspring to survive. The modern human, women in particular, lift very little. Even the amount of time we lift and carry our babies is decreased with the modern conveniences of strollers and vehicles. Loss of muscle mass, also termed sarcopenia, can begin in our 30s and is a syndrome characterized by progressive and generalized loss of skeletal muscle mass and strength. It is strictly correlated with physical disability, poor quality of life, and death. Risk factors for sarcopenia include age, gender, and level of physical activity.[254] Loss of muscle also leads a reduced ability to circulate oxygen as well as to keeping fewer mitochondria and cellular energy assembly lines available to make our precious energy/ATP.[255]

Muscle mass is critical for healthy aging and for weight loss. In my pharmacy, I utilize a body composition machine, the InBody 570, to determine the muscle mass of a patient. This machine uses electricity to distinguish what a body is made of...muscle, fat, and water. Weight and Body Mass Index (BMI) completely fails at discerning these critical measures. On the contrary, the patients of most concern whom I see are "normal" weight, middle-age women. Often, they are women who have starved themselves for years, leading to dangerously low levels of muscle mass. Maintaining independence as we age is often dependent on your ability to function unassisted. My goal is to help you live and age well, and my experience tells me that four things will have us end up in a nursing home: poor nutrition, medication mismanagement (usually too many medications), low muscle mass, and isolation. When one cannot get out of a chair or off the toilet, you will need to live where people can help. All the more reason to really work hard at maintaining or growing muscle. One of the many side benefits of good muscle mass is strong bones. Muscles pull on bones, stimulating them to strengthen throughout life. Good muscle, good bones.[256]

Health Strategy

- Lift heavy stuff!! Focus on muscle growth.

Practice

- Assess your muscle mass through body composition analysis. (Go to Inbody.com/DrKathyHealth to find a body composition assessment near you.)
- Add resistance movement to your day. Stand, squat, make a point to lift things (can of soup, gallon of water, bags of dirt).
- Avoid drive-thru conveniences.
- If you find yourself sitting for long periods, get up every 20 minutes.

- Take the stairs every chance you get.
- Play! Get on the ground, then get up. Throw that ball. Swing that club. Pitch that horseshoe.
- Do yoga, tai chi (isometric resistance training), swim, chop, lift, push, clean, dance.
- WALK!

Run from the Lion

Ancient man rarely ran long distances, and like we said before, never exercised in the way we think of exercise today. Survival often relied on running to eat or avoiding getting eaten! You either ran from the lion and got away, or you did not get away and you got eaten! Pretty straightforward. Our body's ability to respond to that immediate transient threat was critical to human survival and evolution. Those who could flee, survived. As we evolved to be less threatened by man-eating predators, uses of those short bursts of energy might look like chopping wood, grinding corn, or chasing dinner. Today, they're nearly nonexistent.

Current research is beginning to recognize the untapped value of this short spurt of intense activity. With that acute stress response, an almost immediate cascade of chemical reactions (adrenalin, increased heart rate, increased breathing, sugar dumping into your bloodstream) was initiated to help you survive, all to get you away from that lion and keep you alive.

The modern equivalent to running from that lion is termed High Intensity Interval Training. HIIT is a type of workout that consists of short periods of intense movement that gets your heart rate up quickly between intervals of less intense exercise or complete rest. These small, focused and intense bursts of movement have received great attention for their positive impact on metabolic rate, body composition, and energy expenditure.[257] It also does not hurt that they only take a few minutes to do.

> **Health Strategy**
>
> - Get up and move!
> - Incorporate routine short bursts of intense movement throughout your day.
>
> **Practice**
>
> - Dance a two-minute POLKA!
> - Do jumping jacks, jump rope, march in place for 120 seconds multiple times a day.
> - Tabata is a high-intensity interval training that consists of eight sets of fast-paced exercises, each performed for 20 seconds interspersed with a brief rest of 10 seconds.

Hunt and Gather

Until about 12,000 years ago, all humans practiced hunting and gathering for survival. "Hunting and gathering" is a type of subsistence lifestyle that relies on hunting, fishing, and foraging plants (eggs, bugs, honey) for food. For two million years, humans utilized this nomadic search for food as the foundational strategy for life. Because hunter-gatherers did not rely on agriculture, they utilized their mobility as a survival strategy, often requiring an estimated 500 square miles in order to find enough food. It was only about 12,000 years ago, during the Neolithic period, that the shift toward less nomadic, more permanent agriculture-based societies developed. With this shift came a severe reduction in the amount of movement required of humans to survive.[258]

The foundations of human function evolved with this life of

movement. Critical to human existence is the ability to transform chemical energy from your diet into the mechanical energy of movement. As we stated in the "Famine of Chemistry," this production of ATP/energy occurs within the mitochondria, within the muscle, with the delivery of nutrients and oxygen.

Movement, NOT EXERCISE, is critical for human function, specifically the lower intensity, longer duration movement that was foundational to human existence for the first two million years. Recognized today as "Zone 2" training, this moderate intensity (50-70% maximum heart rate) movement produces optimal ATP production, burns fat, and actually stimulates new mitochondrial growth.[259] Turns out the 4-6+ hours of movement that our nomadic, hunting and gathering ancestors required to live is a critical component to optimal human function. Modern research into movement has recognized that *all* humans need this kind of low-intensity, long-duration type of movement for optimal metabolism, even for the most elite athletes. MOVEMENT is critical to life, and much of the dysfunction that plagues modern humans may be due to the severe deficiency of movement (thus the reduced oxygen transport and ATP production).

Modern man no longer has to use his body to live. That is a problem. Getting movement back into our lives *may* look like the modern concept of exercise. The best form of movement is the movement you enjoy and can routinely employ. In a study looking to assess the "best" form of exercise in terms of longevity, it surprised many that tennis/racket sports won with an impressive increased longevity of 9.7 years, while working out in the gym (health club activities) was the least effective, representing an increase in longevity of only 1.5 years. Researchers observed "…the leisure-time sports that inherently involved more social interaction were associated with the best longevity."[260] It may also look like walking to the grocery store, mowing your yard, vacuuming the carpet, playing tag with your grandchildren, or even just chopping your vegetables. All movement counts, and the more fun you have, the better.

Health Strategy

- Build movement into your life.

Practice

- What kind of movement did you love as a kid?
- Track your movement with step-tracking devices. Begin with your baseline bit of movement and work to add more.
- Take that dance class.
- How about an extra lap around the grocery store?
- Get out of that chair (sit to stand) five times per hour.
- Go to the park with a child and play!
- Grow a garden.
- Cook, shred, wash, chop, stir. Put movement into your food.
- Avoid the use of drive-thru convenience when possible. Park your car and go inside.

CHAPTER 15:

Famine of Heat and Cold

"Those who cannot be cured by medicine can be cured by surgery. Those who cannot be cured by surgery can be cured by fire."

~Hippocrates

The coldest I have ever been was in July in the middle of the desert. I will never forget being so cold my teeth hurt! Coldest, you might ask, in the middle of the summer in a desert? I was in Las Vegas, Nevada, in July, in a casino that insisted to air condition the building to what seemed to be a near-freezing level. I could see my breath! My teeth hurt! I literally had to leave and go warm up. I share this story with you to bring to your attention another bit of chaos that our modern existence has brought to our human bodies: the removal of forced temperature variation into our lives. The 20th century brought the incorporation of modern environmental control in the form of air conditioning and heat, driving the modern human to comfortably live inside. No longer were humans living at the effect of seasonal or daily temperature changes. We could now exist in a very comfortable 72 degrees 24 hours a day, 365 days a year (unless you are in a casino in July!). Gone are the physical stresses, adaptations, and repair prompted by seasonal or even daily temperature changes. The increased vasodilation and heart pumping that occurs with heat, and the cellular protection induced by cold, have become less available to us modern humans.

Exposing ourselves to different hot and cold temperatures, though, can be immensely good for us.

A hot sauna, for instance, is good for your heart.

Much like a good workout, a sauna gets you sweaty and increases your heart rate. Even a short sit in a sauna can get your pulse rate up by 30% or more and can get you to pump out a pint of sweat.[261] That rate can double the amount of blood that your heart pumps each minute!

The increased blood flow can ease tension in the joints, relieve sore muscles, and circulate loads of oxygen. More importantly, routine sauna use may have you live longer as it was associated with a very significant decrease in risk of dying from cardiovascular disease![262]

Hot yoga, usually done between 80-100 degrees Fahrenheit, is also known to get your heart pumping, supercharging your respiration and metabolism. The effect can improve circulation to bring oxygen-rich and nutrient-rich blood to your skin cells.[263] Some studies also show that hot yoga programs can boost glucose tolerance in older, obese adults.[264]

On the other end of the spectrum, getting cold has its own set of benefits. Recent scientific interest in cold therapy has shown that cold temperatures provide benefits in reducing depression, anxiety, and stress as well as improving mood and general brain function.[265]

With regard to weight, cold exposure appears to stimulate key positive changes in several important metabolic hormones as well as the production of the very specific metabolically active brown fat.[266] Brown fat, as opposed to white fat, stimulates the metabolism by breaking down blood sugar and fat molecules to create heat and help maintain critical body temperature. Cold temperatures stimulate beneficial brown fat activity.[267]

Could it be the famine of hot and cold is contributing to the modern humans' challenge with weight? I think it is a piece of the puzzle. Begin to embrace opportunities to reintroduce a bit of temperature variation into your life. You do not have to fill up a tub full of ice or go swimming in a lake to get the benefit of cold, though you can do those things. Turning off the hot water and having two-minute cold shower each morning could begin to harness the benefit of cold therapy.

Cold showers are known to improve blood circulation and may also give you a boost of endorphins while decreasing your cortisol levels.[268] The effects of cold include easing sore and aching muscles. Ice baths are also known to help people sleep better, which aids the central nervous system, and are thought to limit the inflammatory response, which can help the body recover and heal.

Certified strength and conditioning specialists say ice baths can also help you face stressful situations better by training your vagus and parasympathetic nervous system.[269]

Health Strategy

- Allow your body to safely experience hot and cold temperatures.

Practice

- Give hot and cold a try.
- Start by simply taking a walk in the elements.
- Try sauna therapy for 3-15 minutes, and see how you feel.
- Try taking a cold shower.
- Try cryotherapy.
- Make an audit of your temperature zones. How often do you experience hot temperatures and cold temperatures?

CHAPTER 16:

Famine of Sunlight

"Here comes the sun."

~George Harrison

Similar to the need for nutrients, oxygen, water, and movement, sunlight is essential for life. Life evolved at the effect of sunlight.

A plant needs sunlight to thrive and produce energy, and we are finding that similarly, we humans need sunlight to thrive. Given our cultural evolution from the plains, to the farm, and into the office, it's not hard to argue we're starved of the life-giving energy of the sun.

The main source of energy to the Earth is radiant energy from the sun. Remember, energy is defined as the ability to produce work, with work being defined as the ability to move things. The sun is essentially a massive nuclear power-plant, radiating huge amounts of life-giving electromagnetic energy out into the universe. Sunlight represents a portion of the electromagnetic energy received on Earth and is grouped based on the level of energy (wavelength) that each category represents.

- **Ultraviolet C** or (UVC) range, which spans a range of 100-280 nanometers (nm). The term *ultraviolet* refers to the fact that the radiation is at higher frequency than violet light (and, hence, also invisible to the human eye). Due to absorption by the atmosphere, very little reaches Earth's surface. This spectrum of radiation has germicidal properties, as used in germicidal lamps.

- **Ultraviolet B** or (UVB) range spans 280-315 nm. It is also greatly absorbed by the Earth's atmosphere and along with UVC causes the photochemical reaction leading to the production of the ozone layer. It can cause sunburn, skin aging, and is required for Vitamin D synthesis in the skin of mammals.[270]
- **Ultraviolet A** or (UVA) spans 315-400 nm. This band is used in cosmetic artificial sun tanning (tanning booths and tanning beds) and in PUVA therapy for psoriasis. However, UVA is now known to cause significant damage to DNA via indirect routes (formation of free radicals and reactive oxygen species) and can cause cancer.
- Visible **range** or **light** spans 380-700 nm. As the name suggests, this range is visible to the naked eye. It is also the strongest output range of the sun's total irradiance spectrum.
- Infrared range spans 700-1,000,000 nm (1 mm). It comprises an important part of the electromagnetic radiation that reaches Earth. Scientists divide the infrared range into three types on the basis of wavelength:
  - Infrared-A: 700-1,400 nm
  - Infrared-B: 1,400-3,000 nm
  - Infrared-C: 3,000-1 mm.[271]

The energy from sunlight stimulates movement and work deep within our cells, fueling the production of our chemical energy (ATP) and other critical processes.[272] The understanding and research of this energy's interplay deep within our cells is explored in the new and exciting areas of study, quantum biology, and photobiomodulation.[273]

One recognized action of sunlight on the human body is the

production of a chemical, commonly termed Vitamin D. Vitamin D is hormone produced by the body as a result of sunlight hitting our skin. I don't know about you, but I rarely find myself running around naked in the sun 12 hours a day as our ancestors may have. Actually, my day job has me hunkered down in an artificially lit cave all day—also known as the pharmacy. I am, as are many of us, lucky to receive 12 minutes of sunlight a day. My life has me chronically challenged to naturally reach an optimal level of Vitamin D.

With the evolution of humans wearing clothes, living inside with artificial light, and applying chemicals that block sun effects, it is estimated that more than 1 billion people (15%) around the world are significantly deficient in Vitamin D.

In the U.S., the estimate is closer to 50% of the population having severe deficiencies in Vitamin D. (Blood levels below the *minimally* accepted level of 25).[274]

Vitamin D, while termed a vitamin, is actually a hormone critical in the optimal function of the human body. Remember, a hormone is a chemical with a job to do. More technically, a hormone is defined as chemical produced in a tissue or organ, with a target action somewhere else in the body. Consider hormones as "chemical keys" seeking out "receptor locks." These chemicals communicate and get stuff done. Such as with the hormone insulin that is produced in the pancreas but works on the cells of the brain (and everywhere else), Vitamin D is produced largely from the skin or is received from the diet and is used to create many cellular results. It turns out that most, if not all, cells in the body have a Vitamin D receptor.[275] You may be familiar with Vitamin D's role in good bone manufacturing, but Vitamin D has a role in many, many critical functions of the body, like proper immune function, thyroid metabolism, and sugar processing.[276]

When we look at Vitamin D's critical role, it is no wonder that low levels of sunlight and Vitamin D production would contribute to many of the chronic dysfunctions or diseases we are currently seeing in our modern "sunless" society. People who are overweight and obese consistently have low Vitamin D levels.[277] Average Vitamin D levels range from 30-100. So, what's best, 30 or 100? The problem is that the range (as with all laboratory ranges) reflects population norms of those tested, not optimal functional levels.[278] These ranges often do not infer optimal or what is optimal for *you*. That fact is important to keep in mind as you look at your laboratory numbers!

Optimal functional Vitamin D levels appear to be much closer to 75nmol/L where reductions in mortality are seen.[279] Luckily, Vitamin D deficiency is a relatively easy thing to assess, recognize, and fix.

Because the body uses Vitamin D to make other chemicals (i.e., cortisol, hormones, etc.), one may get exhausted and deficient during times of high demand, stress, and especially in times of inflammation. Are you deficient? Are you tired, overweight, or have been diagnosed with osteoporosis? Do you have problems with blood sugars being too high? It is important for you to know your Vitamin D levels. The only real way to know for sure is to assess with blood work. Your doctor can order this test at routine exams but may be reluctant to do so due to insurance's reluctance to cover the costs. Do not allow such issues to stop you from receiving this important piece of information. Let the doctor know you will be responsible for the payment. Fortunately, you are now able to access this laboratory information on your own at a moderate expense (Vitamin D for less than $50). (For more information on how to obtain and for comparison costs associated with lab tests it, go to http://www.ultalabtests.com/DrKathyHealth.)

Red Flags

Making sure that you're getting enough Vitamin D might be as simple as spending more time outside in the sun or consuming foods rich in Vitamin D.[280] What if you're doing everything right and your blood work shows you're still low? YOU are the variable. Often, we have low supply because of this lack of sunlight or our diet. But that's not the only cause. Your unique genetics, age, health, and ethnicity can contribute to imbalance, but often the key variables are the demands of your life, with a low supply due to higher demands.

A Vitamin D level of 31 often won't raise a red flag with your physician because it falls within the "normal" ranges. But it should raise a red flag for you.

So, you have gotten blood work, and you are low, now what? We are going to work on supply and demand. Get into the sun! Skin exposure to the sun is the best way to stimulate Vitamin D production. Remember, so much more is happening with the energy from sunlight than just the production of Vitamin D, more than we currently have the capacity to completely understand.[281] It turns out when we shunned the sun to protect ourselves from skin cancer, we may have actually increased our risk of skin cancer. Vitamin D deficiency has been associated with poorer prognosis in those with skin cancer.[282] We need to routinely and safely expose our bodies to sunlight.

It also helps to eat those foods that contain Vitamin D: fish, organ meats, and eggs. Humans evolved eating large amounts of these frequently available foods. (Interestingly, mushrooms are the only plant known to contain Vitamin D.) Over the past 50 years, we've seen a cultural shift away from the sun and away from using the foundational foods through which our bodies evolved. It's harder to get the necessary chemicals to optimally run our human machine. For many, a quality, reliable, and effective pharmaceutical-grade nutritional supplement may be necessary.

Experts now think we may need up to 8,000iu of Vitamin D3 daily to provide our body's necessary support, largely due to the lack of sun exposure.[283] Much larger doses have been used to correct more severe deficiencies. It is important to note that Vitamin D works best with adequate of other critical nutrients, specifically levels of Vitamin K and magnesium. Primitive humans gained large amounts of Vitamin K and magnesium due to their plant-based diet and a robust gut bacterial universe. Modern humans lack both.[284]

Some research has suggested that high-dose Vitamin D supplementation could lead to calcification of arteries, which sounds scary, but that concern wasn't the case when paired with adequate Vitamin K. We are extremely complex chemistry sets, and no drugs or supplements can fully provide us the health and balance that nature has designed. **We must work to get our diet and culture as right as possible.** That being said, I routinely recommend high-quality, pharmaceutical-grade multivitamins containing Vitamin K, combined with Vitamin D 5,000iu daily to support these efforts. Remember before you begin, verify blood levels and discuss these interventions with your health team/chemistry expert. Assess with laboratory again in 3-6 months to see if this regimen is correct for you.

Clearly, the critical role of sunlight is wholly underappreciated and unacknowledged in our modern Western medicine. Vitamin D conversion is just ONE of thousands of potential reactions driven by the energy of the sun in the human body. Many of the chronic diseases plaguing modern humans—obesity, hypertension, depression, cancers, even susceptibility of the flu virus—have been correlated to sunlight deficiency.[285]

Osteoporosis is one such particularly debilitating and often fatal disease where bones are structurally unsound, leading to weakening and breaks. No bone drug, or even Vitamin D replacement, has been shown to come close to the therapeutic impact of a routine dosing of sunlight. In a Japanese study looking at the impact of sunlight on bone over 12 months, 129 elderly, hospitalized, sedentary women were exposed to regular sunlight, while another 129 stayed indoors. The sunlight group increased their bone mass by an average of 3.1%; in the non-sunlight group the bone mass decreased by 3.3%. More importantly, the group who had the benefit of sunlight experienced only one bone fracture, whereas the sunlight-deprived group had six fractures! Sunlight reversed the bone loss![286]

Research into Vitamin D and diabetes (both Type I and II) produces a clear correlation of deficiency to the disease.[287] The Vitamin D hormone plays a significant role in both the production of insulin as well as to the sensitivity of its cellular usage.[288] A 2023 systematic review of prediabetic patients found that Vitamin D supplementation reduced the risk for diabetes in adults with prediabetes.[289] What has not been adequately considered is the role of the sun's ultraviolet energy on our cellular function with regard to these disease states, specifically diabetes. The energy from the sun stimulates your cellular function, not just to increase your Vitamin D levels. Physicians have a difficult time "measuring" the effects of a "dose" of sunlight on your system. This is an exciting area of future study.

The Demand Hormone

The Vitamin D issue is about low supply as well as high demand. Since Vitamin D is a hormone, in times of need, the body will "steal" and chemically convert Vitamin D into other more critically needed hormones/chemicals. The two most critical hormones that can be produced from Vitamin D are aldosterone and cortisol.[290]

Aldosterone is a hormone produced in the adrenals. Its primary function is to keep you upright with the regulation of blood pressure. If you have low aldosterone, you'll have a hard time standing up without passing out due to low blood pressure. If you have too much, as many of us do, it will result in high blood pressure, which causes a whole host of other problems.[291] The right amount is a 24/7 balancing act for your body.

Cortisol is often termed the "master hormone" or "fight or flight" hormone. It is a chemical as critical to human function as are oxygen and water. Cortisol is necessary for many bodily functions like controlling inflammation, blood sugar regulation, metabolism, and most critically "running from a lion."[292] Commonly, we think of cortisol as the "stress hormone." I would like you to consider cortisol as the "demand hormone." One could have very low levels of "stress" in your life and still require large amounts of cortisol. Many of us may not consider our lives "stressful" but experience very demanding lives. Even events as wonderful as getting married, having a baby, or thriving in a career require great production of cortisol from the body. Eating a modern diet low in nutrients and high in processed, inflammatory "foods," requires big reserves of cortisol to survive. In the pharmacy world, cortisol is a powerful steroid anti-inflammatory medicine. The same medication we would give you for say a swollen knee, or a bad poison ivy rash, your body will produce in response to a high-sugar, high stress life. In times of high demand, the body will prioritize production of cortisol, aldosterone, and other critical hormones in order to keep you going and keep you from getting eaten by that lion. As a strategy for survival, the body may strategically stop making less critical hormones (i.e., testosterone, estrogen, thyroid, Vitamin D, etc.) and steal these reproduction hormones to turn them into the more critical master "survival" hormones.

Beware of where you are putting your body at a disadvantage. Too little sunlight and our crazy demanding, modern life is a recipe for chaos. Low supply/high demand means you don't have enough chemicals to run your machine properly. Remember, your primitive brain will ensure that you survive. It will adjust the system in order for you to stay warm and breathe. This survival may not be particularly comfortable, or desired, but it is survival. Obesity, depression, hypertension, fatigue, anxiety…what if these were the appropriate results of this survival? What if these were the symptoms and not the real problem?

What are the demands on your system? How well stocked are you in the supplies needed by your system? Asking these questions are the keys to your health. Consider your body's demands like browsers on your computer, each requiring energy, each requiring a response. The more you have up, the slower and less efficient your computer works. The same is true for your body.

Health Strategy

- Optimize your chemistry with sunlight.

Practice

- Challenge yourself to spend a little bit more time outside in the sun.
- Sit out on your porch while you drink your morning coffee.
- Eat lunch on a picnic table or restaurant patio.
- Read a good book on a park bench.
- Take a morning or evening walk while listening to a podcast or your favorite tunes.
- Work in the garden.
- Working from home? Take that laptop outside to work.

Brain dump: Write down everything going on in your life. Journal all of the apparent demands of your life: work, kids, relationships, economics. Write down all of the issues and all of your concerns. The task is not to do anything about them (that can come later)—just get it down on paper.

What are your current symptoms of a system that is challenged? Tired, anxious, cold, irritable, sleepless? They are potential clues as to how your system is having to adapt. Complete the medical symptom questionnaire (MSQ) at drkathysays.com/MSQ.

CHAPTER 17:

Famine of Darkness

*"It was the possibility of darkness that
made the day seem so bright."*

~Stephen King

It was not long ago that all human existence was determined by the cycle of the sun—12 hours of light, and 12 hours of darkness, more sun in the summer, less sun in the winter. These on/off cycles, also termed circadian rhythms, represent physical, mental, and behavioral changes that follow a 24-hour cycle. Deep within every cell of our body we have "cellular clocks" scheduling and regulating the immense amount of work needed to keep you going.[293]

The presence and, maybe more importantly, the absence of light are powerful environmental triggers influencing our clocks. It is during this absence of light, and subsequent sleep, that the body's maintenance and repair systems kick into high gear. (The presence and absence of food seems to also be a critical driver of our clocks' cellular processes as well.)

Both sunlight and its regulation of the critical hormone melatonin are key components of sleep. Melatonin is a hormone produced deep within the brain from the primitive pineal gland. During the day, sunlight sends the signal to the pineal gland, blocking melatonin production. During the darkness of night, the pineal gland is stimulated to produce melatonin, beginning the start of sleep and many of the subsequent repair processes.

Melatonin is key for sleep, prevents cancer, is a powerful antioxidant, and is important in the production of many other critical chemicals needed in the body. One chemical you may be familiar with is the neurotransmitter serotonin.[294] Lack of melatonin due to too much light will cause major disruption in serotonin production and could be a contributor to much of the mental and physical health challenges we see today.[295] Lack of sleep and the subsequent lack of melatonin production could indeed be contributing to your health and weight issues.[296]

Modern life has really messed up this primitive cycle. Ever since the advent of electric lighting, we have light available 24/7. While Wall Street may enjoy that we can be much more productive, the body is massively challenged by the lack of darkness, the lack of melatonin, and subsequent lack of this necessary programmed sleep, rest, and repair.

The body is so sensitive to light that melatonin may be suppressed not only with the light received through the eyes, but also with light received exclusively through the skin, including the eyelids. Yes, your skin is a light- and darkness-detecting organ! Turns out those personal computing devices, smart phones, night-lights, and other modern light-emitting electronics are powerful hormone disrupters![297]

According to Harvard Health, some studies have linked exposure to light at night—whether you're working the night shift or scrolling on your smart phone—to obesity, heart disease, and diabetes.

Blue Light

Blue light, the kind that typically comes from electronic screens, can suppress melatonin production for about twice as long as other kinds of light, according to Harvard researchers. Blue light can come from fluorescent and LED lightbulbs—you know, the kinds that are good for the environment. Research shows that the old incandescent lightbulbs we grew up with are better for our sleep patterns, even if they are worse for the environment.[298]

Correcting this famine should begin with the intentional reintroduction of darkness and sunlight into your life. Sunlight in the morning and darkness in the evening. Morning light provides the body with the raw materials and the cues needed to make nighttime melatonin, as well as the production of good amounts of Vitamin D. The proper mix of daylight and darkness is the beginning to getting the sleep your body *needs* to properly function.

Ideally, we should build offices and schools with care to encourage exposure to natural sunlight, as is the case with some European building standards.[299] We should get children outside to play multiple times a day.[300] Outdoor classrooms and offices should be structured into our day. And then as the sun begins to set, we should bathe ourselves in the darkness that is coming. Minimize the amounts and types of light to which you are exposed, making all effort to experience the light and darkness of the day. In order to protect ourselves from blue light, we can avoid looking at bright screens for two or three hours before we go to bed. If you work a night shift or use computers for much of the day, consider getting blue light blocking glasses. Those steps must be foundational.

Health Strategy

- Optimize your circadian rhythm by optimizing your exposure to sunlight and limiting artificial light.

Practice

- Audit the light in your life! How much sunlight are you exposed to during the day?

- When the sun goes down, how much artificial light are you exposed to? Artificial light includes interior lighting, cell phone/computer/TV screens, and more. Can you adjust the blue light settings on these devices? Can you avoid such devices altogether?
- Try putting away all electronic devices one hour before you go to bed and see what kind of a difference it makes in your sleep patterns.

Adults typically need between 7-9 hours of sleep each night. Take note of how much time you're setting aside for sleep—and if you are actually sleeping through the night! If you notice you aren't getting at least seven hours of sleep, and that your sleep is restless, these are some strategies you can use to improve your sleep.

1. Stick to a sleep schedule, even on the weekends. Go to bed and get up at the same time each day.
2. Cut back on caffeine, alcohol, and nicotine. All three can negatively impact your sleep.
3. Avoid exposure to blue light screens before going to bed.
4. Avoid daytime naps if you can.[301]
5. For some, I'd recommend a quality melatonin supplement. Supplementation of 1-3mg at bedtime may be useful in efforts to support a challenged system.

CHAPTER 18:

Famine of Sleep

"Sleep is the best meditation."

~Dalai Lama

Sleeping is really, really important—breathing while you sleep is critical. I have observed nothing in my 30 years of practice as crisis-provoking for the body as low oxygen (see Famine of Oxygen, Chapter 13). The body and brain **freak out** and adapt if they sense not enough oxygen. Just like the panic you would feel if could not get a breath under water, the brain reacts in many adaptive ways when oxygen is low.

Some adjustments are slow over time (i.e., slower metabolism, reduced temperatures, fatigue, low initiative, etc.); some are immediate (i.e., panic/anxiety, elevated heartbeat, etc.). As I mentioned in that chapter, oxygen is life. Now consider oxygen at night.

When we sleep, our automatic systems run the show. The night shift begins the enormous task of cleanup and repair. Deep, slow breaths, full relaxation, blissful dreams—until there is a crisis. Dips in oxygen at night (as well as dips in blood sugars) create an all-out "red alert" for the brain. When the brain senses low oxygen, a shift is triggered from the hormones of rest and recovery to the complex hormonal "fight or flight" survival response. Adrenalin is dumped into the system, sugar from the liver is dumped into the bloodstream, the heartbeat increases, leptin, ghrelin, and insulin are secreted in response to the sugar and adrenalin, and you are brought out of that deep, restorative sleep into a light sleep, or you wake up in order to breathe. (You might also notice that this waking is when you feel a need to go to the bathroom.) All of those reactions happen because the automatic systems were not able to keep you breathing well. Low oxygenation during sleep, also termed sleep apnea, is a big threat, a big contributor to chronic health challenges, and obesity. When hormones (adrenalin, cortisol, etc) and nighttime blood sugars are elevated, one can find it almost impossible to lose weight. This nighttime oxygen/hormone roller-coaster may contribute to your gaining weight, and then the weight you have gained can make the low oxygen/sleep apnea worse! [307] It is a nasty, vicious circle.

For many, it may feel like you are worn-out tired upon awakening. For some, it may look like weird elevations in your heart rate during the night. For some, the only symptom may be your inability to lose weight. In some ways, you have chemically run a marathon in your sleep. Little of the restorative, healing processes that **must** occur during sleep will be able to occur if nighttime oxygenation is a problem. Your brain spends all night making sure you do not DIE! If those conditions describe you or someone you love, spend all of your effort in getting your sleep assessed and getting your sleep improved. Your life may depend on it.

Health Strategy

- Optimize nightime breathing and blood sugar.

Practice

- Answer these questions:
  - Do you snore?

- Do you dream?
  - How often do you wake up when you need to without an alarm?
  - Are you exhausted upon awakening?
  - How often do you *need* caffeine to get through the day?
  - How many times do you wake to go to bathroom at night?
- Assess your sleep with a home sleep apnea test or app.
- Bring the results to your physician for possible assistance in nighttime breathing.
- Sleep on your side.
- Oxygenate well during the day with lots of movement.
- Consider continuous blood-glucose monitoring in an effort to identify low/high blood sugar swings during the night. **(drkathysays.com/cgm)**

CHAPTER 19:

Famine of Connection

"Only by restoring the broken connections can we be healed. Connection is health."

~Wendell Berry

After 40 years of studying chemistry, what I know is there is no more powerful chemistry for health and human function than the chemistry of love and connection. Love heals. That declaration may seem a bit strange coming from a science-based clinical pharmacist, but the "science" speaks for itself. The chemistries created by the body with love and connection are powerful, healing, and necessary for human existence.

Your brain is programmed and wired to survive. This "wiring," also known as your nervous system, is exquisitely and sometimes frustratingly designed to anticipate and respond to threats. Your biology is programmed through generations of your ancestors' past experiences in order to predict and prepare you for what is around the corner that might eat you. It is programmed to fight. It is programmed to flee. It is programmed to hide. It is programmed to survive. (If you have not noticed, most of what our brain predicts never ends up happening, getting us all worked up for nothing!) Your genetics—the biology handed to you at birth—have evolved to prepare you for the environment into which you emerged in order for you to survive. This turning on or off of your genetics, also termed epigenetics, is a function of the environment in which your brain/body finds itself. It is estimated that your physical function is the result of 30% genetics and 70% environment![302]

In response to an environmental stimulus, the brain will orchestrate the production and release of powerful chemicals that drive you to respond. These chemicals, sometimes referred to as stress hormones, are very powerful chemicals. Cortisol, catecholamines (adrenalin, noradrenalin, dopamine, serotonin, etc.), insulin, and vasopressin are just a few of the chemicals produced as a stress response and orchestrated in order for you to respond and survive. For our ancestors, the threats were pretty straightforward and temporary. We ran from the lion, got away, and the stress hormones went down, or we got eaten and our hormones went down! For modern humans, the stresses never seem to go away. We are always running from the lion and overproducing these powerful, and in chronic, high amounts, toxic chemistries. The impact of these stress response chemicals coupled with the fact they seldom go down contributes to much of the chronic health challenges present today.[303]

Humans cannot survive alone. We are a social species hardwired for connection. Evolutionarily, our safety and our survival depend on the presence and cooperation of others. From your first heartbeat, your nervous system develops in response to the environment it encounters. The human nervous system takes decades to fully develop, each neurological wrung creating the foundation for the next. The development of the brain and body is critically dependent on internal (nutrients, toxins, hormones, etc.) and external (social stimulation, warmth, chaos, prenatal, etc.) environmental cues. The warm, safe, cuddled, well-fed, and nurtured (low stressed) infant develops a resilient, well-coordinated, optimal nervous system. Stressors in our early life can lead to abnormalities in our neurological development, the subsequent stress responses, and our lifetime health and well-being.[304]

For all things living, life is hard. Humans have never, ever survived alone. Survival is the complete and total focus of your brain. All of your body's processes, thoughts, cravings, and chemical and emotional reactions are exquisitely orchestrated through the lens of survival. **(IF** survival is handled, reproduction is your body's next priority. And for all of you parents out there, once you have children, a big part of your brain (annoyingly) will forever be concerned about *their* survival.)

We are a social species who evolved, survived, and thrived relying on the secure connection of others for safety and sustenance. Our primitive brains knew that our "tribe" had our back. Our brains knew that there would be food, protection, and comfort in the difficult world.

Just as our brain sends fight or flight chemicals in times of "threat," our brains produce very different and powerful chemistries during times of "no threat." Where there is love and connection, there is perceived safety. There is also oxytocin. Oxytocin is the primary chemistry produced during this "love/safety response" and has been directly linked to improved health and longevity. Implicated in defending against some of the established "hallmarks of aging," oxytocin is powerful medicine in reducing oxidative stress, inflammation, free radicals, cancer-causing mutations, and shortening of telomere (distinctive structures found at the ends of our chromosomes).[305] When your brain is loved and safe, it is able to repair and renew. Love heals and makes you live longer!

Humans are hardwired for connection, hardwired for belonging. From our first heartbeat our nervous system's "wiring" develops in response to the connection from the nourished warmth, sound (heartbeat) and safety of our environment/mother.[306] Once born, our nervous system explodes in its growth. As adults, humans create approximately 750 neural connections a day. For the infant, it is estimated that they are creating a million neural connections per second![307] When a baby is born, only the lower regions of the brain are fully developed at birth, and much of the higher, more complex levels of the brain will not become fully developed for decades. Infant brains are exploding with its interaction from the world. An infant's brain is sampling its environment in order to activate the genetics necessary for survival. The development of the brain (and subsequent body) is critically dependent on internal (nutrients, toxins, hormones, etc.) and external (social stimulation, warmth, chaos, etc.) environmental cues. Even the touch and cuddling of a baby affect how they grow and develop and leave marks on their DNA.[308] The first months and years of human development lay a delicate foundation for future function, each developmental wrung of the neurologic ladder being critical to the proper development of the next. A warm, loving, calm, nurturing, well-nourished, connected environment creates the critical cues for optimal neurological development. Lack or disruption of these cues will critically alter this neurodevelopment. The latter is the core understanding of the dysfunction created by adverse childhood events.[309]

The last 100 years have presented a profound cultural shift in how humans live, resulting in a profound deficiency in human connection and safety. Modern cultural shifts in how we live have created an epidemic of isolation and contribute to our chronic mental and physical health crisis.[310] No longer do we live multi-generationally or in clans. We are culturally encouraged to be "independent," and often, being alone is a badge of honor. That state is not okay with our brain. We were never designed to be alone. Critical to the health of your body are loving and secure relationships, which are not limited to an intimate partner and can include the neighbor you wave to, the gang at the coffee shop, a pet, or your favorite relative. It could be the moms at your children's school or the volunteer group that cleans up the local park. Wherever these healthy and supportive relationships come from, they are critical for creating the most impactful chemical conditions for health.

The Recipe

What's the recipe for good health? Oxygen, sunlight, water, good food, and love. The proper combination is simple, but it's definitely not easy. Getting these simple chemistries right is difficult, not because of you, not because you are weak or undisciplined. It is difficult because we live in a culture that makes it very, very difficult. We live in a culture that produces disease, one that advertises toxic food, celebrates independence/isolation, and profits greatly on your "dis-ease." In addressing these critical chemistries, you may find yourself going against many cultural norms. You may cook and eat that vegetable instead of running through that drive-thru. You may take a walk as opposed to spending the evening surfing technology. You may choose to spend your evening as a volunteer at the local food bank or with friends. It may seem that you are going against what "society" would steer you to do. That's okay, you are worth that effort. Surround yourself with the tools and team to support your being well, and if you are putting any chemistry into your machine, make sure a pharmacist is on your team. You are never stuck as the human you are, and you are worth whatever it takes to have the health you want to live the life you want.

Health Strategy

- Build Connection.

Practice

- Volunteer in an area that brings you joy.
- Take a class.
- Spend time with others at your local coffee shop, or library.
- Teach others something you are good at.

CHAPTER 20:
Famine of Safety

"The brain creates the world, but early in life the world creates the brain."

~Gabor Mate, MD

The brain is tasked with having the body survive its environment. From the earliest moments of life, external inputs are being funneled through the brain and creating biological understanding, responses, and strategies for survival. Challenges faced by the nervous system may even result in a strategic response that is passed on to future generations.[311] The research around early childhood stress is fascinating and striking. Drs. Vincent Filetti, MD and Robert Anda, MD are responsible for the groundbreaking research called the Adverse Childhood Experience Study (ACE Study). In their work, adverse childhood experiences have been directly correlated with physiologic changes and disease. ACE science now includes the ways that toxic stress in childhood affects children's brain development, the short- and long-term health effects of toxic stress, the epigenetics ("above the genes") of how toxic stress alters gene expression, and how genes are passed on from generation to generation, as well as research in resilience.

I had the great fortune to meet and visit with Dr. Filetti about his groundbreaking work. In our conversation, I commented that it is almost like the brain is self-medicating in its seeking of external relief. "That is exactly what the brain is doing!" he exclaimed. "We doctors had to deal with our own arrogance. What we thought was the problem (addiction, obesity, depression…) was actually the brain's solution."

In my experience, unresolved, unacknowledged early childhood trauma can appropriately make you sick and make you fat. I am reminded of a visit from a lovely 53-year-old patient, M. M. was a fit medical practitioner who booked an appointment to discuss hormone balance. She was a very talented practitioner and was was seemingly very healthy. I was humbled by her faith in me and began to ask what I could do to support her. She mentioned fluctuations in her hormones, but ultimately disclosed that her biggest challenge and the reason she was seeing me was for assistance with an unrelenting, life-long depression. No matter what she had tried, a blanket of depression continuously wrapped her. She mentioned that she was at her best when she was working a critical situation (code blue) in the emergency room.

Understanding the research of adverse childhood events, I began to dig a bit deeper. I noticed she had an accent. Even with my limited knowledge, I recognized the accent to be Eastern European or possibly Russian. She confirmed that she was indeed from Russia. Thinking about how growing up in 1970s Soviet Russia might have been, I asked, "Was there alcoholism in your family?" "Oh, yes," said M. "My father was a raging alcoholic, and my earliest memories were of my mother holding me between her and my father so he would not beat her."

Could you imagine?

For M. and many children developing in worlds of high external stress or neglect, the brain and body are literally created in a pool of excessive stress chemistries. The body responds (survives) to this "normal" by increasing hormones and receptors, altering neural development and the brain architecture, creating smaller or larger areas of the brain. The body will adapt to this "normal," and if not addressed, may result in increased incidents of pathology, chronic disease, and possibly early death.[312] What is so interesting about the research is that many who are asked about these stressful childhoods do not perceive them as stressful. They just see them as normal. Because they have no other reference, or because the environment was common to others, stressful childhood environments are often not noted as being stressful or "abnormal." Chronic poverty, abuse, absent parents, low-nutrient/toxic foods, drugs and alcohol, and war are sadly, in many lives, the norm.

I shared with M. the research surrounding the ACE Study, the impact of childhood adversities on the growing brain, as well as how her body had so miraculously supported her survival by preparing her to survive in a high-stress environment.[313] The biggest clue was how good she felt when she was in the stressful (high-stress hormone adrenalin) emergency room situation. Experiencing excessive fight or flight hormones was her "normal." Her 'low-stress' adult life away from the ER contrasted with a very different set of experiences that her growing brain/body had been prepared for in childhood. The result of this low-adrenalin life contributed to a relative 'deficiency' in these critical chemistries.

She was relieved by this insight, but for me it was not enough. I asked her, "But what do we do to help you not feel depressed?" She had already tried many pharmaceutical and botanical strategies with little success. "Do you like to exercise?" I asked, thinking that medicating with exercised-induced "stress chemistries" might help.

She did like to exercise and said she could definitely do more. "Medicating" with morning exercise—in her case, running—could intentionally generate a strategic increase in these "stress chemistries", replicating the increased levels that had occurred as a fearful child. Running in the morning and actively resting in the evening could begin to strategically support her system. In addition, her understanding of the role that chronic childhood stress is playing in her life can be extremely freeing and be the beginning to her "re-parenting/re-programming" this dynamic.[314]

Our brains create strategies in order for us to survive life's challenges. These survival strategies are complex biochemical, emotional, and behavioral patterns unconsciously developed from conception in response to our environment. How you perceive and respond to the world may still be influenced by your three-year-old self! These developmental strategies are not bad...on the contrary, they helped you to survive. They may not, though, be the best strategies today in order to achieve optimal health and vitality. Because they keep you prepared for those prior issues and circumstances, they may not be the best strategies to help you achieve what you want today! They can be extremely difficult to release.

I have a well-developed survival strategy of independence. Early in life, my young brain determined that to "survive" I needed to not bother my parents and be good at everything without their help. I became very good at anticipating needs and proactively solving problems. This very valuable survival skill made me a great independent pharmacist. This strategy, though, will not create the culture of health that I so want for our grandchildren, and it is lonely. I WILL NEED HELP! I cannot do this alone. I am learning to recognize the help that I need. I am learning to accept contribution. I am learning to quiet the internal dialog that says "I am a bother." I am learning to ask for help. These new and often unfamiliar, uncomfortable strategies are critical to my producing the new results I wish for my life.

The good news is we are never stuck with these survival strategies or their impacts. The work of Bruce Perry, MD, shows us that not everyone experiences the negative effect of childhood adversity. Those with resilience appeared to be protected from many long-term negative effects. Resilience is defined as the capacity of individuals to navigate their way to the resources they need and to negotiate for those resources to be provided in ways that are meaningful.[315] As Masten and Powell write: "Resilience refers to patterns of positive adaptation in the context of significant risk or adversity."[316] Often, resilience is seen as an individual trait—you either have it or don't. That belief is incorrect. Resilience is a skill. It may be helpful to reimagine resilience as a function of the environment in which you find yourself. A resilient "culture" is one filled with supportive resources utilized in navigating stressful times. Crafting a life rich in these supportive resources (LOVE) and utilizing them during times of need consciously builds our resilience muscle and has a direct, positive impact on our health. This "re-parenting," as I termed it with M., is available and valuable to all of us regardless of our early life.

Health Strategy

- Build your resilience.

Practice

- Take the ACE questionnaire. Discuss it with a health care provider who understands its impact.
- Write down the story of your life. What do you remember? Where did you feel loved and connected? When did you feel scared?
- How resilient is your life? Audit the supportive resource you have access to.

Remember, there is nothing wrong here. YOU HAVE SURVIVED! The goal is to identify the survival strategies in place that may no longer be optimal.

Seek out the support of a behavior health professional in understanding the impact that adverse childhood experiences may play in your life

Follow my colleague and life coach extraordinaire David Leifeste, LPC (DavidLeifeste.com) for new, supportive strategies. His book *The Possibility of You. The OASIS Secret to a Wonderful Life* is a gift to give yourself or someone you love.

CHAPTER 21:

Famine of Support

"Loneliness and the feeling of being unwanted is the most terrible poverty."

~Mother Theresa

Being alone is as bad for your health as smoking 15 cigarettes a day.[317]

Our primitive development and survival depended on a secure attachment to the people around us and on an ability to quickly assess those who loved us from those who wanted to kill us. Our connection to other humans—that basic sense of belonging and safety—impacts the function of our human machine, both as infants and as aging adults. Being connected to other humans is as necessary as oxygen and nutrition are for health. The modern human is in an epidemic of isolation, and it is killing us.

Both actual and perceived social isolation are associated with early death.[318] Being the pharmacist/chemist, I tend to try and understand what chemically is happening in the body that could cause the illnesses in order to assist my patients. Isolation falls into the category of what I call "stress pharmacology." Our magnificent machine evolved to anticipate and respond to threats in order to stay alive and reproduce. We have evolved an amazing sensory organ, the brain, exquisite in its ability to sense, predict, and respond to threat. The brain has an uncanny ability to predict and prepare for the threat that "might" be coming around the corner. Once a threat is perceived, the brain triggers powerful chemical chains of events. Adrenalin, cortisol, insulin, glycogen, glucagon, and aldosterone are just a few of the chemicals produced in order for us to react, in order for us to survive. These chemicals have us FIGHT, FLIGHT, or FREEZE in order to survive threat. They are POWERFUL, and in large, persistent doses, TOXIC chemicals. For most living animals (and for our ancestors), when a threat approaches, all of those chemicals are dumped into our system, and we respond. We either get away, and the chemicals go down, or we get eaten and the chemicals go down. Either way, the effects of the powerful chemicals were transient.

For modern humans, threats—real and perceived—never go away. All the current concerns (the mortgage, the bad boss, inflation, crazy political leadership, etc.) are made more intense by the 24/7 nature of media and technology. As discussed in previous chapters, cellular starvation (not enough of the chemistries needed to run the cellular machines) is a *huge* threat to survival. Add to this chaos the disruptive toxic burden that modern chemicals have on our cellular machines. They are real chemical threats to our survival. *Then* we have to deal with the chronically elevated "fight or flight" stress chemicals. Unlike modern humans, primitive man never worried about what was happening on the other side of the planet.

Worse yet, we are often marketed to and manipulated to take action (buy) through fear. We must vote a certain way, send our children to a certain school, buy a certain type of clothes, drive a certain car in order to belong in order to "survive." It is crazy! And that sensory organ designed to keep you alive by predicting and recognizing these threats—the brain—has an uncanny ability to "make up" possible threats that may not even be real! Many of our chronic diseases are the result of or made worse by the unrelenting stress chemicals produced in response to this threatening world and account for an incredible 75% of all doctor visits.[319]

Health Strategy
• Build Support

Practice
• Build your Partner in Health team. You are in charge of your team. Anyone can be on this team (do not forget the value of a great hair dresser or barber to impact how you feel!). In addition to the physician and a pharmacist, often a physical therapist, chiropractor, nutritionist, a farmer, a psychologist, a massage therapist and a large friend network are wonderful contributors to a supportive team and your good health.
• Own a pet. If this is not possible, consider volunteering at a shelter or to watch a friends pet when they go out of town. The benefits are both ways.
• Volunteer with others in your community to impact an issue important to you. Rock babies at the local hospital, pick up trash in the park, read to children at the local school...do something you love to the benefit of others.

CHAPTER 22:
Famine of Relationships

"Despair often breeds disease."

~Sophocles

Never in the history of humanity have we been so alone to navigate the world. Smaller families, cultural changes in how we work, shop, and connect have forever altered our baseline human interactions and thus, our human physiology. Our modern world has arranged our lives to *appear* to not need each other for survival, which wasn't the case for our ancestors. No longer do we "need" our neighbors to help build the barn, to raise children, or to help hunt and gather. Yet, nothing could be further from the truth.

Do you have friends or relatives that you can count on when in trouble? Do you feel safe walking alone at night in the city or area that you live? How satisfied are you with the freedom of choice in your life? How easy is it to get around (public transport) in your area?[320] For many modern humans, the answer to such questions begins to reveal just how separated and disconnected we are from each other. Modern technology has made things worse. With that small computer we carry around and 24/7 social media, we have the "illusion of connection." The stress chemistries produced with what actually is isolation is making us sick.

Health Strategy

- Increase positive relationships.

Practice

- Engage with others around a hobby or passion.
- Audit your likes and dislikes. Dive into learning something new. Often you will find yourself with new and interesting people.
- Acknowledge those around you that make a difference for you and the world. Let them know.
- Seek out or become a coach or mentor.
- Join a support group or take a class.

CHAPTER 23:

Famine of Hope

"Once you choose hope, anything's possible."

~Christopher Reeves

We all are familiar with that feeling of fear where all we want to do is run or hide. Many of my patients come to me figuratively "curled up under a rock" or self-medicating in order to survive the threats of their life. Tired, depressed, irritable, overweight, and medicated may be appropriate response strategies for surviving the perceived and real threats of our modern world. Unlike the lizard that might temporarily crawl under the rock to avoid threat, modern humans never seem to get away from the threats of our lives.

One solution to our concerns often employed by the brain is self-medication. As stated by Dr. Filleti, alcohol, drugs, food, gambling, and work are just a few ways the brain seeks to relieve the discomfort of this chemical chaos. Unfortunately, the short-term relief that these "strategies" provide are at the cost of long-term health and survival. The impact of the chemicals from the addictive "strategy," coupled with the impact of the stress chemicals, contributes to chronic disease and the current decline in life expectancy.[321] Termed "Diseases of Despair," they represent an increasing category of deaths attributed to drug abuse, suicide, and alcoholism. The situations associated with despair-related disease include financial distress, lack of infrastructure or social services, deteriorating sense of community, and family fragmentation.[322] The impact of those factors could probably be a whole book, and that prospect is profoundly sad to me.

According to the Centers for Disease Control and Prevention, U.S. life expectancy has been declining for years. Sure, as more data about COVID-19 comes out those numbers could be skewed even further, but the data tells a sad story. Deaths caused by suicide and drug overdoses have skyrocketed. In 2018, the most recent data available, suicide was the 10th leading cause of death in the U.S., accounting for 48,344 deaths. According to the American Foundation for Suicide Prevention, there were an estimated 1.4 million suicide attempts in the same year.[323] In 2018, even before the COVID-19 pandemic, the CDC named overdoses, especially of opioids, a key contributor to the shortening U.S. life expectancy. A crazy, stressful, toxic world, with fewer connections to share life's burdens or give us a hug, is killing us.

Connection with Community

In this day and age, we often feel we are more connected than we actually are. Modern social media is a big part of the problem. With that little electronic box in our palm, we have the "illusion of connection." We have thousands of "friends" but no one next to us for that smile, hug, laugh, or cry that generations of humans took for granted. A couple of generations of children have been raised in a culture deficient in meaningful connection and touch, and they are not doing well. According to the American Psychological Association, adolescents and young adults are experiencing striking increases in mental health issues than in previous years, including psychological distress, major depression, and suicide attempts. Dr. Jean Twenge, PhD and author of the book *iGen* speculates that the rampant use of digital media is part of this frightening equation. She argues this form of media alters how young people communicate as well as how much young people sleep. At a time when young, developing nervous systems require the consistent inputs from safe, nurturing connections, (and optimal nutrients!) many grab or are handed an electronic screen.

"Technology is robbing the soul of our communities," stated my colleague David Leifeste, LPC. As a 40-year therapist and executive coach, David observes, "Western culture seems to have the tendency to overcommit, whether that is the children's schedule or the lifestyle demands. People think, 'if my kids are going to be successful (i.e., survive), they need to be in three sports, need to be doing well academically, and must be well-connected socially.' Everyone has so many places to be. The tail of the schedule is wagging everyone's priorities. Some connections happen in these scheduled activities, but often they are very task-oriented and not about intimacy."

It is not just our imagination or David's observation that our busy life is interfering in our connection to community. One study reveals about 3:5 people in 2019 agreed to take on more than they possibly had time for. That same study showed that another 1:5 had reached their limit and could not commit to doing any more. The study included both personal and professional commitments. Being over-stretched led to additional stress, worry, anxiety, overwhelm, and defeat. About 44% of participants reported that because of their long to-do lists, they only felt "really present" (i.e., connected) only half of the time. A whopping 37% said they rarely or never felt present. That kind of overcommitment creates tremendous physical demands and chaos for our bodies and for our lives. On the other extreme, living alone, being physically isolated, or just lonely has been shown to increase your risk of depression and early death![324] We are in a nasty, vicious, culturally sponsored cycle that is killing us.

How do we interrupt this cycle? "I remind people that one of the most rewarding forms of connection can be giving back to others," David said. "There are a lot of needs in every community...whether you take time to help at a shelter for animals or for people, or you just do something nice for your neighbor, it provides an immediate rush of good feelings." David also recommends finding an organization or group of others centered around something you are interested in—things that are aligned with your interests, your needs, and your personality. If you live alone, consider getting a roommate—no matter your age! When David works with his patients to get them out of "survival mode," he likes to point out that what you like and enjoy are God's clues to yourself. It is in that moment of enjoyment that your chemistry is calm...love is present and where healing happens.

It is important that we slow down! It is important that we connect. A really impactful place to begin is with our food. It used to be that we hunted, gathered, and prepared our food. We had to *really* work to get that meal ready. It took time and effort. It was in that time and effort that our body began to prepare for the chemistries heading its way. Then there was the sitting down and enjoyment of the meal that often many people at the table had contributed to providing. These days, we drive thru to buy and scarf down already highly processed and often toxic chemistry called "food." Often this 'toxic and deficient food-like substance,' is half way through the gut before it is even thoroughly chewed or before the body is chemically ready to begin to digestion.

Slow down. Process your own, real food. To the greatest degree possible, connect to your food. Grow it, shop for it, wash it, chop it, cook it, enjoy it...process your own food. Find opportunities to share a meal with other humans. Connect, digest, absorb, and breathe. It sounds simple. In our current culture, it may be simple, but it is definitely NOT EASY. It is very countercultural to be healthy.

Health Strategy

- Craft a culture that produces health.

Practice

- With each exercise in this book, we have been examining the culture/environment in which you live and the health you have as a result. YOU can craft a new culture. New chemistries, new relationships, new actions, new environments will create new results. It may feel very odd...even difficult for a while. Soon these new actions will feel normal. It is currently very countercultural to be healthy. It is worth the effort. YOU are worth the effort. Lean on your Partner in Health Network to support and be supported in creating the health you wish.

CHAPTER 24:

Famine of Touch/Love

"To love someone is to strive to accept that person exactly the way he or she is, right here and now."

~Fred Rogers

Warm, safe, and cuddled, the human infant thrives. So does the human adult!

A component of "stress pharmacology" that is largely ignored by modern medicine is the impact and power of the "positive" chemistries produced with touch and connection. Dopamine, oxytocin, vasopressin, serotonin, norepinephrine are a few powerful chemicals produced when love, connection, fun, and safety are present.[325] After 30+ years as a practicing pharmacist, I have learned there is no greater intervention, no more powerful chemistry for healing than love. LOVE HEALS. (Second to that is the power of food!)

Opposite to the damaging impact of chronically elevated "fight, flight, or freeze" chemistries, the "love, connected, and safe" chemistries produce profound positive health effects. Longevity studies have consistently found tremendous positive health impacts from a mother's love, rich social connections, and intimate relationships.[326] Fun, love, happiness, safety, and, yes, health, is a function of our relationships. One study found a remarkable

50% reduction in death with the presence of strong social relationships![327] NO DRUG has ever been prescribed that can come close to that kind of outcome (and many that we dispense try!). Seldom recognized in the often-mechanical and transactional world of modern medicine, the role of love is largely unstudied and often "pooh-poohed." It is difficult to quantify and measure. It is difficult to dispense through the mail! The business of medicine and insurance cannot profit on something as intangible as love. Catastrophically, in modern health care—or more accurately, modern disease care—if it is not diagnosable, measurable, and "prescribable," it has *no* value.

A critical way that humans (and animals) communicate love and connection is through touch. For humans, touch signals to the brain the presence or absence of "safety and connection." Unfortunately, cultural changes in human existence have prompted us to touch less, which is in stark contrast to our primitive ancestors who literally wore their children so they did not get eaten! The infant was physically connected to the parent 24/7. A crying infant was a beacon for animals, so the child was carried near the breast and encouraged to feed for comfort as well as safety. The infant brain is literally being programed with every interaction as it samples the environment to determine the best developmental strategies. Touch has been shown to correlate to improved brain development, health, and survival of the infant.[328] Modern cultural expectations of independence and self-reliance, coupled with technology, have fostered changes in how modern human parents live, work, and play. Modern parenting strategies diverged greatly from our nomadic ancestors, resulting in the separation of the infant/child from the mother and forever changing the developing neurology and genetics.[329] "Never hug and kiss them, never let them sit in your lap" became the 20th century's "scientific" strategy for "successful" modern parenting. Generations of parents separated themselves from their developing infant in a well-intentioned effort to do the "best" for their child. This disassociation has contributed to the catastrophically-wrong environment for optimal human neurologic development. From conception on, many of these changes have reduced the opportunity for positive touching and have caused many of us to be deficient in the positive chemistry of touch. Our Western culture, where independence is prized, is particularly conditioned to "touch less." Lack of connection and lack of touch leads to very disordered human development.[330] Being with other humans creates a level of perceived safety and helps to reduce and minimize the perceived and real threats in life.

The evidence is very clear: If you love and are loved, you live longer with less disease.[331] Patients who had strong social relationships and received empathic health care were healthier and had better outcomes.[332] My interacting, connecting, smiling, encouraging, and—dare I say—LOVING my patients in my small independent family pharmacy has produced health for my patients and for myself! The time that your physician and pharmacist used to take to understand your worries and your world was a cornerstone in building a loving, trusting, and empathetic therapeutic relationship that helped you be well. That attention, that time, has been systematically removed by the "business" of health care.

Connection with Self

At some point in our childhood, the brain makes up who we have to "be" to survive. This identity or what I call the "survival self" is a carefully crafted brain response to the environment and survival. As we grow and receive environmental cues, we attempt to understand and predict the external world in our effort to be safe. The strategies that bring this perceived safety and understanding make up this survival identity. For me, I became a "good girl." As the seventh of eight children to older, depression-era parents, I developed a "survival self" that was very quiet, of little trouble, and asked little of my parents. I created as little chaos as possible in order to survive. I "hid" a lot in an attempt to avoid negative energy. I learned to be uber competent, compliant, and independent. It is no accident that I became an independent (isolated) pharmacist! I became very good at figuring things out, anticipating the needs of those around me, and providing solutions. I looked externally as to whom I needed to *be* in order to survive. I became a servant. Those are the perfect skills for the independent pharmacist that I have become. Unfortunately, though, I have come to realize that my primitive, childhood survival strategies of complying and being alone are today not sufficient in providing me the life my 56-year-old self really wants (and deserves).

As I stated earlier, I want a long and intimate relationship with my daughters and grandchildren. I really WANT to dance at my granddaughter's wedding. I want to age well, have physical strength and vitality. I want a brain that works well. I want to function well for a long time. I want to contribute to their life and not be a burden. I want Abby to be at that wedding, enjoying the health we have created and laughing a bit at her crazy mom. I WANT Abby, Emma, and their children (and your children) to live in a world that would support them in being well, to support them in having healthy children. I REALLY WANT our grandchildren to be born into a world where their health, not their disease, is prioritized. I want them to be born into a world where they will be healthy. I want a world where people do not need medications. I am clear that my old, comfortable survival strategies of compliance and isolation are not what is needed to make these "wants" happen. New, uncomfortable strategies like asking for help, being bold, and being loud may (will) be needed to have this world emerge.

What do you want? For many of us, wanting is "hushed" out of us by five years old. Young children want everything. Many of us are told "NO" enough to become scared into not asking. In our effort to survive, we begin to lose the ability to want, lose the ability to dream. "Wanting" is the destination. I want energy, peace, fun, joy, love. I want a culture that produces health. I want to dance and share love at my granddaughter's wedding. What do you want?

What strategies did your brain employ—or is still employing—to become your "survival self?" In our attempt to find peace and safety, many of the survival strategies under which we evolved may actually be very maladaptive and do not produce the results we really want. Workaholism, gambling, overeating, substance abuse, isolation, and individualism are a few of strategies we may use to soothe the "survival self." My adaptive strategy of being compliant and independent did help me survive and become a successful pharmacist, but may hinder me in creating the culture of health that I so want. My aversion to seeking help from others may not be the most effective strategy in achieving my dreams. Remember there is no "good" or "bad" here, only what works and what does not work in achieving your "destination." Who is your "created self?" What do you want? These questions and their thoughtful answers will set your course.

What does your "internal dialog" tell you about who "you" are and what "you" should do? No matter what you say to yourself, about yourself, your brain is always listening—it is the "internal dialog." The impact of these internal thoughts are powerful drivers of our health. Your brain will produce stress chemistries when it perceives life as stressful and scary. It will also produce very different chemistries when it perceives that same life as a safe, fun, challenging adventure. That lion coming at you…are you thinking, "Oh, no, I am going to get eaten? Or do you think, "Look at that magnificent animal?" Which perception is right? For many, our early neurological development or programming resulted in a positive internal dialog, for others a negative one. The good news is that "YOU ARE NEVER STUCK AS THE HUMAN YOU ARE!" Our internal dialogs can be "reprogrammed" and carefully crafted to produce the results we want.

Health Strategy

- Know and love thyself.
- Connecting with your "self" is important. (Maybe I should say connecting with your "selves" is important.)

Practice

- Begin to listen and write down those internal thoughts.
- Make note of some of the familiar patterns/strategies that have had your life work well.
- What are familiar patterns that have had your life not work as well as you would like?
- What do you love? What are your likes, dislikes, interests, dreams?
- What do you want?
- Who is your "survival self?" Begin to recognize when your "survival self" is running the show. Make note.
- Who is your "created self?"
- What survival strategies do you find exciting in others?
- What strategies do you dislike or make you uncomfortable? Make note.
- Be kind, gentle, and nurturing toward yourself.
- Seek out a team practitioner skilled and focused on supporting you along this journey.

CHAPTER 25:

Famine of Purpose

"The meaning of life is to find your gift. The purpose of life is to give it away."

~Pablo Picasso

If the brain can't see the future, if it does not have something to look forward to, it freaks out. The brain is a receiver tasked with your survival. It is always trying to anticipate when that lion will jump out from around that corner. We have survived for as long as we have by being able to predict and avoid the worst. The brain has been programmed over millions of years to keep you alive! The truth—and the problem for many—is that most of what we dream up, all of those terrible things we fear could happen, never happen or may not actually be a threat. That loud noise on television, that looming mortgage payment, being alone…are not an actual threat to your life, not like the lion was to your ancestors. But you still process those things through your survival receiver (brain), causing powerful stress chemistries to release. Increased heartbeat, blood pressure, blood sugar, and, yes, weight gain all produced in order to be safe and "run from that lion."

If the distractible brain cannot see a future path, it will make up the "safe" path complete with all of the "dangers" that you should avoid. It is important that we know ourselves and give our brain understanding and direction. A purpose is a declared path for the brain to understand and follow. David notes, "Every morning when you wake up, your brain is waiting for its marching orders. If we do not wake up with a sense of purpose and hope beyond survival, we are in trouble." Having a sense of purpose, he states, is critical so that there is a sense of anticipation and hope. That goal gives your brain the direction it needs so that your choices will sync up and lead you where you want to go.

According to the American Psychological Association, hope is associated with increased happiness, better academic achievement, and even reduced risk of death. Hope has been further defined as having three key parts—goals, agency (action), and pathways. In other words, purpose is our destination, hope is the plan and process to get there. Both are important to your journey. Knowing yourself well enough to know that in any given situation who you are and why you are here helps your brain respond more calmly and get you where you WANT to go.

WHAT DO YOU WANT? This is the start to your journey. I want you to have a great life, and health is foundational. Early on with my patients, I sit down with them and ask them to begin to dream, to begin to articulate what they want for their future. There will be challenges on this journey…hard challenges. You live in a culture designed to make you sick, to make you fat. It is difficult to be healthy, but it is not hard *because* of you. You live in a culture that makes it very hard to be well, and as you may begin to recognize, it is very countercultural to be healthy. When you understand that bias, it should make you a bit angry. Use that anger. Use that anger to do the hard things to be well. Take that walk. Cook that meal. Drive past the fast food. Use that energy to make the challenging investments in your health. YOU HAVE THE ABILITY TO RESPOND. It is in each response that you will direct your future.

Health, and life, is a journey. It is never static and seldom on course. Imagine yourself, your body, as that airplane or a sailboat. Some of us are

747s, some Piper cubs, some Learjets. The systems in each plane being in good repair and well fueled are important to all "flights." We do not wait to check these things out or maintain the machine when we are in the air! We do not allow parts to wear out before we replace. We always use the correct fuel. We proactively anticipate needs and aggressively maintain the vehicle for optimal function. Anything less could be disastrous.

A well-maintained vehicle sitting at the airport has little value. The value is in the vehicle's ability to travel. Key to the journey is the destination. I am in Tulsa, and I want to go to New York City. Knowing the destination, determining a course, and then programing in the travel coordinates are fundamental to beginning your journey and arriving at your intended destination. Where are you going? Where do you want to go?

Purpose is your proposed destination in life. Purpose is the future you create to live toward. You are here, and you want to be there. For me, my purpose—my stated destination—involves twerking at my granddaughter's wedding…having a long, intimate relationship with my daughters and future grandchildren. Fundamental to that goal and my life is creating a culture that has myself, my husband, my children, and my world be well. That objective sets my course every day.

A stated purpose beyond the default human survival is critical for your journey, providing the coordinates, the marching orders for your machine. Where do you WANT to travel to in life? Who do you WANT to be? What prompts you to get out of bed in the morning?

I once asked a patient of mine if flights are ever always on course. He was a pilot, so he was uniquely qualified to answer. "NEVER," he stated, "we are *always* course-correcting depending on the conditions of the flight." Rest assured, the journey to your destination will never be a straight line. LIFE will blow you off course. Pandemics, deaths, injuries, births…the winds of life will demand that you assess, adjust your sails and course-correct. Critical to those corrections is your being clear in where you want to go.

My hope is that the information in this book will support you in your journey. Please, please, please realize YOU HAVE SURVIVED! Your brain, body, and spirit (and those of your ancestors) have survived in the most miraculous of ways and often in the most unbelievable circumstances. Yes, you may carry extra weight. You may have experienced changes in your psychology, but you are here, and often with little direction or help. YOU ARE NEVER STUCK AS THE HUMAN YOU ARE. Your body has appropriately adjusted and adapted to the environment of your life. You and your body are to be celebrated and, now, supported. Throughout this book, my hope is that you are assessing your environment, your culture, and the myriad of challenges that your body may be navigating. Insufficient nutrition, toxic foods and drugs, nutrient deficiency, low oxygen, poor gut absorption, excessive demands, deficient sunlight, toxic water, lack of connection, early trauma…what have been and are your challenges? As you explore, discover, and address the "famines" challenging your system, new actions, new directions, a new life will emerge.

This is important. Begin to shift your thinking away from shame and blame. In and of themselves, choices are neither good nor bad. There is just what those choices produce in your unique body and life. Do these choices aim you where you want to go? Shame or blame are useless (and actually can produce toxic stress chemistries!). The same applies to foods. Personally, I would eat donuts everyday if it worked for my body. I am clear that donuts are toxic for my brain, however, so I strategically avoid them. It is important to listen to what each choice, thought, bite produces in your unique machine. There are "foods" that cause us to be sick or produce certain results that we may or may not want. Does that food or thought or action make you anxious? Upset your stomach? Cause your joints to hurt? Improve your sleep? Give you energy? Correlating what happens with each input is important. All are clues on your journey.

With each assessment, each correlation, you are learning to navigate your unique health. You will be creating a new environment for your body to exist in…a new culture…ultimately creating the health you want to live the life you want.

Health Strategy

- Create a Culture of Health.

Practice

- Clarify your purpose, wants, and dreams.
- What you want is *the* hardest question, but the one that sets the destination! Allow yourself to DREAM! "I WANT_____!"
- What do you NOT want?
- Where are you currently heading?
- What famines are you experiencing?

Ask yourself these questions:

- How often do you see friends and family—people who bring joy into your life (not on social media, or by phone, but in person)?
- Who is on your health team (flight crew)?
- How many smiles do you send out to others every day?
- How much time do you spend alone daily?
- Volunteer at a place that makes the difference you want to make.
- Go for a walk where other people are walking.
- Learn something new with others. Take an art class, go to the library.
- Learn to polka! (Fun, movement, and people!!)
- Play with your grandchildren.

CHAPTER 26:

NOURxISH!

"People never change because of threat or duress. Never. They change because they see something that makes their life seem valuable enough to start moving toward a life worth living."

~Robert Downey Jr.

It is my hope that through this book you will begin to recognize and embrace that your magnificent body has survived and is serving you. YOU HAVE SURVIVED! You have survived severe cultural mis-nourishment/malnourishment. You have survived cultural shame, trauma, and disconnection. You have survived a culturally-driven sedentary life. You have survived toxic chemicals marketed as food. You have survived a medical system that depends on your being sick. You have survived a profoundly damaging environmental/cultural shift in how humans live. The obesity that has for many been a source of pain and disease was your body taking care of you. Is obesity problematic? Yes. Is it the problem? No. Obesity is the symptom. Look to where acceptance (love) is missing in your life. Did you feel accepted as a child, young adult? Do you accept yourself now? Are you accepted by your physician? Being accepted and being loved is life for humans. For many of us, acceptance is hard to find. Our society does not accept obesity, and neither do we, for that matter. We have been shamed—from family, from physicians, from society, from ourselves. You must not allow your health to be determined by insurance companies, your doctor, or the narrative of Wall Street. You are valuable. You are unique. YOU have the power to be well.

I want you to have a great life, and I know health is foundational to it. If we don't have the right chemistry to run our body, there will be appropriate consequences. Our current medical system is NOT designed to evaluate you on an individual level, even though *you are* **THE ONLY YOU**. Our current medical system is NOT designed to help you course-correct and prevent, delay, or reverse the onset of disease. Our current medical system is not designed to assist you in being well. Truly being well will be up to you.

Your brain, body, and spirit (and those of your ancestors) have, in the most miraculous of ways and often in the most unbelievably traumatic circumstances, survived. Yes, you may carry extra weight. Yes, you may have experienced changes in your psychology, but you are here, and often with little direction or help. YOU ARE NEVER STUCK AS THE HUMAN YOU ARE. Your body has appropriately adjusted and adapted to the environment of your life. You and your body are to be celebrated and, now, supported. Throughout this book, my hope is that you are assessing your "environment, your culture, your famines" and the myriad of challenges that your body may be navigating. Insufficient nutrition, toxic foods and drugs, nutrient deficiency, low oxygen, poor gut absorption, excessive demands, deficient sunlight, toxic water, lack of connection, early trauma… what have been and are your challenges? What is your body telling you? As you explore, discover and address the "famines" challenging your system, new manageable actions, new directions, a new life will emerge. New environment. New culture. New results. New life.

Throughout this book, I listed a variety of health strategies and exercises to help you get to know yourself better, learn what famines you may be experiencing, and to begin to journey in a new direction. My challenge to you now is to take the next step. What is the easiest, first thing for you to do? Take that step. Then take another. You can do this. I am rooting for you!

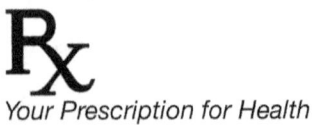
Your Prescription for Health

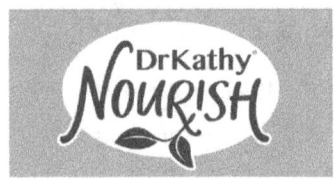

Spicy Rotisserie Chicken Soup

1 lb. onions, diced
1-2 lbs. carrots, diced
1-2 lbs. celery, diced
2 T. olive oil
2-4 T. garlic, chopped
1 T. dried parsley or 1 bunch fresh, chopped
1 t. salt
freshly ground black pepper

Cook on medium heat in a large stock pot until veggies are soft.

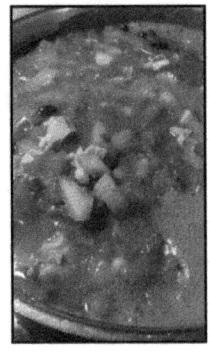

Add:
5 cans Rotel tomatoes with green chilies
1-14.5 oz. can diced tomatoes (more of this & less Rotel for less spicy)
2-4 cans black beans, rinsed and drained
6-8 c. chicken bone broth (see recipe below)
3-4 c. rotisserie chicken, diced

Bring to a light boil, reduce heat to low. Simmer for at least 1 hour to bring out flavors. Refrigerate leftovers.

Rotisserie Chicken Bone Broth

Place the bones of a rotisserie chicken into a large pan and cover with water. Bring to a boil. Reduce heat and cover. Simmer for at least 1 hour. Strain through a colander to remove bones. Refrigerate broth to separate fat.

During this high virus season, fortifying yourself and your family with this powerful "medicine" is essential. This is my delicious prescription for health!

MEDICAP PHARMACY
130 S Main St
Owasso, OK 74055
918-274-1737
drkathysays.com

Prescriber: *Dr Kathy*
Kathy M. Campbell, PharmD

Dr Kathy Says...

Food is the chemistry of life. It is the foundation to health and if lacking, the foundation of disease. No matter how hard medicine tries, there is no substitute for the healing power of real food. Looking back over my 35 years of studying chemistry and the human body, an article I came across in 2001 sparked a deep, lasting curiosity and forever changed the way I practiced pharmacy.

The remarkable study from the journal Chest was titled, "Chicken Soup Inhibits Neutrophil Chemotaxis in Vitro." The researchers concluded, "The present study, therefore, suggests that chicken soup may contain a number of substances with beneficial medicinal activity." Yes, this study had confirmed what grandmothers throughout generations have known very well - chicken soup is indeed good medicine.

Fortify, Enjoy and Be Well!

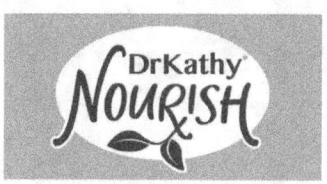

DrKathy Health ©2020

Acknowledgements

This book—my life, really—is the product of many people loving and supporting me. First on that list, is my husband Royce Campbell. Thank you, Royce, for your unending devotion, love, support, and for your gentle way of making it all work out. To my daughters, Emma and Abby: Thank you for so generously sharing your mom with the world, and for the love, joy, and fun you bring to 'DrK.' Nothing is more rewarding than seeing you two embrace and live your lives.

To my parents, Paul and Dolores Brooks. Thank you for teaching me that hard work will always get you closer to where you want to go (Mom) and that you can't worry and fish at the same time (Dad). You modeled for me a life of contribution, love, and growth.

To Patrick Turner. You have always been my biggest fan. I cannot imagine who I would have become if you had not interrupted my knitting in the dorm that Friday night so long ago. Your 40 years of unwavering, unconditional love and friendship has supported me in creating the most wonderful life. Thank you for loving and valuing me and for teaching me to do the same for myself.

To my Cornett "framily," Sue, Gayellen, Angela. Thank you for embracing me into your lives so many years ago. Always being there to laugh and love me, in good times and bad.

To my friend, mentor, and sponsor, Beverly Schaefer, RPh. Thank you for leadership and vision and for always creating a safe, loving, supportive space for me to grow.

To my book team, both at Book Launchers and my local coffee shop: Thank you for your gentle persistence, confidence, and support in birthing this book. Your professionalism and encouragement have been critical its completion, especially in navigating the massive distraction of one pandemic.

To my pharmacy support team, Tonya, Gena, Jacque, Sam, Dena, Amina, Travis…thank you for all that you are and all that you do. Every day you show up and live our mission to assist our community in having great lives. In good times and bad, through health or PBM theft, or a pandemic, you, like small pharmacies around the world, show up and care. Thank you for caring for me.

Finally, to my friends and patients in the community of Owasso, OK. For 32 years I have learned from you. You have so generously placed your trust and health into our hands. It is through our journeys that the foundations of this book were laid. Your friendships and faith have provided me the most magnificent life of service and purpose. Your love heals me every day. Thank you for so generously including me in your great lives.

To learn more about how to navigate our modern famines—whether that's through a lifestyle mentoring group, getting discounted lab information, learning what supplements might help you, and more—connect with me at **drkathysays**.com.

Endnotes

1. Phelan, S., D. Burgess, M. Yeazel, W. Hellerstedt, J. Griffin J, and M. van Ryn. "Impact of weight bias and stigma on quality of care and outcomes for patients with obesity." Obesity Reviews 16, no. 4 (2015): 319-326, doi: 10.1111/obr.12266.
2. Ibid.
3. Ibid.
4. "Constitution of the World Health Organization," accessed March 31, 2023, https://apps.who.int/gb/bd/PDF/bd47/EN/constitution-en.pdf.
5. Ibid.
6. Felix F. Lillich, John D. Imig, and Ewgenij Proschak, "Multi-Target Approaches in Metabolic Syndrome," Front Pharmacol 11 (2021): 554961, doi: 10.3389/fphar.2020.554961.
7. Hannah L. Kushnick, "Medicine and the Market," AMA Journal of Ethics 17.8 (2015): 727-729. https://journalofethics.ama-assn.org/sites/journalofethics.ama-assn.org/files/2018-06/joe-1508.pdf
8. Ann Gibbons, "The Evolution of Diet," National Geographic online, accessed April 4, 2023, https://www.nationalgeographic.com/foodfeatures/evolution-of-diet/.
9. Quin Li et al., "Obesity and Hyperinsulinemia Drive Adipocytes to Activate a Cell Cycle Program and Senesce," Nature Medicine 27 (2021): 1941-1953, doi: 10.1038/s41591-021-01501-8.

10. Briana Pobiner, "Meat-Eating Among the Earliest Humans," American Scientist 104 (2016): 110-112, doi: 10.1511/2016 .119.110.
11. Travis Hay, "Commentary: The Invention of Aboriginal Diabetes: The Role of the Thrifty Gene Hypothesis in Canadian Health Care Provision," National Library of Medicine, 28 (2018): 247-252, doi: 10.18865/ed.28. S1.247.
12. Komlos, J and M Brabec, "The Trend of BMI Values by Deciles of US Adults, birth cohorts 1882-1986" NBER Working Paper (2010): 16252.
13. Jean Rankin et al., "Psychological Consequences of Childhood Obesity: Psychiatric Comorbidity and Prevention," Adolescent Health Medicine and Therapeutics 7 (2016): 125-146, doi: 10.2147/AHMT.S101631.
14. David M. Cutler, Edward L. Glaeser, and Jesse M. Shapiro, "Why Have Americans Become More Obese?" Journal of Economic Perspectives Summer 2003, https://www.brown.edu/Research/Shapiro/pdfs/obesity.pdf.
15. "Julia Child's Kitchen." National Museum of American History, accessed on April 1, 2023. https://americanhistory.si.edu/food/julia-childs-kitchen.
16. Leah Binkovitz, "FOOD: An Edible Exhibit Examines Our Many Culinary Cultures," Smithsonian Magazine, November 20, 2012. https://www.smithsonianmag.com/smithsonian-institution/food-an-edible-exhibit-examines-our-many-culinary-cultures-138576448/.
17. Cristin E. Kearns, Laura A. Schmidt and Stanton A. Glantz, "Sugar Industry and Coronary Heart Disease: A Historical Analysis of Internal Industry Documents," JAMA Intern Med. 176, no. 11 (2016): 1680-1685, doi: 10.1001/jamainternmed.2016.5394.
18. "Which Is Worse for You: Fat or Sugar?" Cleveland Clinic: Health Essentials September 10, 2019, https://health.clevelandclinic.org/which-is-worse-for-you-fat-or-sugar/.
19. "Junk Food and Your Health," healthdirect January 2021, https://www.healthdirect.gov.au/junk-food-and-your-health.
20. Joel Fuhrman, "The Hidden Dangers of Fast and Processed Food," American Journal of Lifestyle Medicine 12, no. 5 (2018): 375-381, doi: 10.1177/1559827618766483.

21. Heather Rogers, "The Functional-Medicine Matrix," Experience Life online, accessed April 6, 2023, https://experiencelife.lifetime.life/article/the-functional-medicine-matrix/.
22. Heather Alexander, "What Are Macronutrients?" June 2020, https://www.mdanderson.org/publications/focused-on-health/what-are-macronutrients-.h15-1593780.html.
23. "What Are Macronutrients?" last modified June 1, 2021, https://www.webmd.com/diet/what-are-macronutrients.
24. Lizzie Streit, "Micronutrients: Types, Functions, Benefits, and More," last modified August 3, 2020, https://www.ncbi.nlm.nih.gov/pmc/articles/PMC6379287/.
25. Suzanne Wakim and Mandeep Grewal, "Nutrients," LibreTexts, last modified June 8, 2022, https://bio.libretexts.org/Bookshelves/Human_Biology/Human_Biology_(Wakim_and_ Grewal)/04%3A_Nutrition/4.2%3A_Nutrients.
26. "Whole Foods," NYC Health, accessed April 1, 2023, https://www.nyc.gov/site/doh/health/health-topics/whole-foods.page.
27. Forrest Hooton, Giulia Menichetti, and Albert-László Barabási, "Exploring Food Contents in Scientific Literature with FoodMine," Scientific Reports 10 (2020): 16191, https://doi.org/10.1038/s41598-020-73105-0.
28. "Showing Food Garlic," FooDB, accessed April 1, 2023, https://foodb.ca/foods/FOOD00008.
29. Albert-László Barabási, Giulia Menichetti, and Joseph Loscalzo, "The Unmapped Chemical Complexity of Our Diet," National Diet 1 (2020): 33-37, https://doi.org/10.1038/s43016-019-0005-1.
30. "Only 1 to 10 Adults Get Enough Fruits or Vegetables," CDC Newsroom, last modified November 16, 2017, https://www.cdc.gov/media/releases/2017/p1116-fruit-vegetable-consumption.html.
31. "Lightweight Skeletons of Modern Humans Have Recent Origin," John Hopkins Medicine, last modified December 22, 2014, https://www.hopkinsmedicine.org/news/media/releases/lightweight_skeletons_of_modern_humans_have_recent_origin.

32 Allison Balogh, "The Rise and Fall of Monoculture Farming," last modified December 13, 2021, https://ec.europa.eu/research- and-innovation/en/horizon-magazine/rise-and-fall-monoculture- farming.

33 Ibid.

34 "How Industrial Agriculture Affects Our Soil," FoodPrint, last modified December 1, 2021, https://foodprint.org/issues/how- industrial-agriculture-affects-our-soil/.

35 Rita Bia, Roberta Farina, and Elena Brunori, "Family Farming Plays an Essential Role in Preserving Soil Functionality: A Study on Active Managed and Abandoned Traditional Tree Crop-Based Systems," Sustainability 13, no. 7 (2021): 3967, https://doi.org/10.3390/su13073967.

36 Henry Ford and Samuel Crowther, My Life and Work (Garden City, NY: Doubleday, Page & Company, 1922).

37 "Vitamin Deficiency Test," ADA online, last modified September 22, 2022, https://ada.com/micronutrients/vitamin-deficiency-test/.

38 Jacob Dunn and Michael H. Grider, "Physiology, Adenosine Triphosphate," last modified February 23, 2023, https://www.ncbi.nlm.nih.gov/books/NBK553175/.

39 Tatiana El Bacha, Mauricio R. M. P. Luz, and Andrea T. Da Poian, "Dynamic Adaptation of Nutrient Utilization in Humans," Nature Education 3, no. 9 (2010): 8, https://www.nature.com/scitable/ topicpage/dynamic-adaptation-of-nutrient-utilization-in-humans- 14232807/.

40 Sabzali Javadov, Andrey V. Kozlov, and Amadou K. S. Camera, "Mitochondria in Health and Diseases," Cells 9, no. 5 (2020): 1177, doi: 10.3390/cells9051177.

41 Jacob Dunn and Michael H. Grider, "Physiology, Adenosine Triphosphate," last modified February 23, 2023, https://www.ncbi.nlm.nih.gov/books/NBK553175/.

42 Ibid.

43 Bernard Cuenoud et al., "Brain NAD Is Associated with ATP Energy Production and Membrane Phospholipid Turnover in Humans," last modified December 16, 2020, https://www.frontiersin.org/articles/10.3389/fnagi.2020.609517/full.

44 Tingting Hou et al., "Mitochondrial Flashes: New Insights into Mitochondrial ROS Signalling and Beyond," The Journal of Physiology 592, no. 17 (2014): 3703-3713, doi: 10.1113/jphysiol.2014.275735.

45 John N. Meyer et al., "Mitochondria as a Target of Environmental Toxicants," Toxicological Sciences 134, no. 1 (2013): 1-17, https://doi.org/10.1093/toxsci/kft102.

46 Xianhua Wang et al., "Mitochondrial Flashes Regulate ATP Homeostasis in the Heart," eLife 6:e23908 (2017), https://doi.org/10.7554/eLife.23908.

47 "Micronutrients for Your Mitochondria!" accessed April 1, 2023, https://caltonnutrition.com/micronutrients-for-your-mitochondria/.

48 "Metabolism Overview," LebreTexts online, April 13, 2020, https://med.libretexts.org/Courses/American_Public_University/APUS%3A_An_Introduction_to_Nutrition_(Byerley)/APUS%3A_An_Introduction_to_Nutrition_1st_Edition/06%3A_Energy_Metabolism/6.02%3A_Metabolism_Overview.

49 Katy McLaughlin, "Aerobic Respiration," last modified August 25, 2020, https://biologydictionary.net/aerobic-respiration/.

50 Massimo Bonora et al., "ATP Synthesis and Storing," Purinergic Signal 8, no. 3 (2012): 343-57, doi: 10.1007/s11302-012-9305-8.

51 Susan Gallaghar, "What Can Hunter-Gathers Teach Us about Staying Healthy?" last modified April 19, 2021, https://globalhealth.duke.edu/news/what-can-hunter-gatherers-teach-us-about-staying-healthy.

52 Jacob Dunn and Michael H. Grider, "Physiology, Adenosine Triphosphate," last modified February 23, 2023, https://www.ncbi.nlm.nih.gov/books/NBK553175/.

53 Caroline R. McKeown and Hollis T. Cline, "Nutrient Restriction Causes Reversible G2 Arrest in Xenopus Neural Progenitors," Development 146 (2019): 20, doi: 10.1242/dev.178871.

54 Kelly J. Gibas, "The Starving Brain: Overfed Meets Undernourished in the Pathology of Mild Cognitive Impairment (MCI) and Alzheimer's Disease (AD)," Neurochemistry International 110 (2017): 57-68, doi: 10.1016/j.neuint.2017.09.004.

55 Brent M. Kious, "Hunter-gatherer Nutrition and Its Implications for Modern Societies," Nutrition Noteworthy 5, no. 1 (2002). https://escholarship.org/content/qt4wc9g8g4/qt4wc9g8g4.pdf?t=krne6g.

56 Monica Herald, "Why Are the World's Biggest Animals Plant Eaters?" last modified January 20, 2020, https://www.worldatlas.com/articles/why-are-the-world-s-biggest-animals-plant-eaters.html.

57 Celia Smoak Spell, "There's No Sugar-Coating It: All Calories are Not Created Equal," last modified November 4, 2016, https://www.health.harvard.edu/blog/theres-no-sugar-coating-it-all-calories-are-not-created-equal-2016110410602.

58 Terezie Tolar-Peterson, "Not All Calories are Equal – A Dietitian explains the Different Ways the Kinds of Foods You Eat Matter to Your Body," The Conversation online, accessed April 3, 2023, https://theconversation.com/not-all-calories-are-equal-a-dietitian-explains-the-different-ways-the-kinds-of-foods-you-eat-matter-to-your-body-156900.

59 Alexandra Sifferlin, "'Eat Less, Exercise More' Isn't the Answer for Weight Loss," Time online, last modified June 3, 2014, https://time.com/2809007/eat-less-exercise-more-isnt-the-answer-for-weight-loss/.

60 Sousana K. Papadopoulou et al., "Exercise and Nutrition Impact on Osteoporosis and Sarcopenia. The Incidence of Osteosarcopenia: A Narrative Review," Nutrients 13, no. 12 (2021): 4499, doi: 10.3390/nu13124499.

61 "Dementia From Nutritional Deficiencies," Dementia.org, July 2, 2015, https://www.dementia.org/diet-induced-dementia-nutritional-deficiencies.

62 Yvette Brazier, "What is nutritional-deficiency anemia?" last modified December 6, 2019, https://www.medicalnewstoday.com/articles/188770.

63 Molly Burford, "9 Vitamin and Nutritional Deficiencies That May Cause Depression," last modified August 25, 2021, https://psychcentral.com/blog/nutritional-deficiencies-that-may-cause-depression.

64 "The Connection Between Obesity and Nutritional Deficiencies," Long Island Laparoscopic Doctors, last modified May 15, 2020, https://journeytothenewyou.com/blog/the-connection-between-obesity-and-nutritional-deficiencies/.

65. "How Poor Nutrition Contributes to Fatigue," Optimal Performance Medicine, accessed April 3, 2023, https://www.optimalperformancemedicine.com/blog/how-poor-nutrition-contributes-to-fatigue.
66. Chakell Wardleigh, "Does Dieting Make You Anxious?" accessed April 3, 2023, https://selecthealth.org/blog/2021/07/does-dieting-make-you-anxious.
67. Anna Guerdjikova and Harold C. Scott, "Dangers of Dieting: Why Dieting Can Be Harmful," Lindner Center of HOPE, accessed April 3, 2023, https://lindnercenterofhope.org/blog/why-dieting-can-be-harmful/.
68. Jason Howland, "Mayo Clinic Minute: How to Ease the Itch of Mosquito Bites," last modfied July 6, 2022, https://newsnetwork.mayoclinic.org/discussion/mayo-clinic-minute-how-to-ease-the-itch-of-mosquito-bites/.
69. "Celiac Disease and Lactose Intolerance," Beyond Celiac, accessed April 3, 2023, https://www.beyondceliac.org/celiac-disease/related-conditions/lactose-intolerance/.
70. "Foods that trigger overeating," Piedmont, accessed April 3, 2023, https://www.piedmont.org/living-better/foods-that-trigger-overeating.
71. Steven J. Russell, "Continuous Glucose Monitoring," National Institute of Diabetes and Digestive and Kidney Diseases, last modified July 2017, https://www.niddk.nih.gov/health-information/ diabetes/overview/managing-diabetes/continuous-glucose-monitoring.
72. Malin E. V. Johansson, Henrik Sjövall, and Gunnar C. Hansson, "The Gastrointestinal Mucus System in Health and Disease," Nature Reviews Gastroenterology & Hepatology 10 (2013): 352-361, https://www.nature.com/articles/nrgastro.2013.35.
73. Ryan D. Rosen and Ryan Winters, "Physiology, Lower Esophageal Sphincter," last modified March 17, 2023, https://www.ncbi.nlm.nih.gov/books/NBK557452/.
74. "Gastroesophageal Reflux Disease," Mount Sinai online, last modified February 6, 2022, https://www.mountsinai.org/health-library/diseases-conditions/gastroesophageal-reflux-disease.
75. "What Is GERD?" UCI Health, accessed April 3, 2023, https://www.ucihealth.org/medical-services/esophageal-disease/gerd/what-is-gerd.

76. Sylvie Tremblay, "What Minerals Contract a Muscle?" SFGATE online, last modified December 6, 2018, https://healthyeating.sfgate.com/minerals-contract-muscle-6293.html.
77. "Hypochlorhydria," Cleveland Clinic online, last modified June 27, 2022, https://my.clevelandclinic.org/health/diseases/23392-hypochlorhydria.
78. "The Best and Worst Foods for Acid Reflux," University Hospitals online, last modified April 16, 2014, https://www.uhhospitals.org/blog/articles/2014/04/best-and-worst-foods-for-acid-reflux.
79. "What Is Hypochlorhydria?" WebMD, last modified November 15, 2021, https://www.webmd.com/digestive-disorders/what-is-hypochlorhydria.
80. "Small Intestinal Bacterial Overgrowth (SIBO)," Mayo Clinic, accessed April 4, 2023, https://www.mayoclinic.org/diseases-conditions/small-intestinal-bacterial-overgrowth/symptoms-causes/syc-20370168.
81. Perry A. Frey and George H. Reed, "The Ubiquity of Iron," last modified July 30, 2012, https://pubs.acs.org/doi/pdf/10.1021/cb300323q.
82. "Iron," ACS Publications online, last modified April 5, 2022, https://ods.od.nih.gov/factsheets/Iron-Consumer/.
83. Nazanan Abbaspour, Richard Hurrell, and Roya Kelishadi, "Review on Iron and its Importance for Human Health," Journal of Research in Medical Sciences 19, no. 2 (2014): 164-174, PMID: 24778671; PMCID: PMC3999603.
84. Ibid.
85. "World Prevalence of Anaemia 1993-2005," WHO Global Database on Anaemia, last modified 2008, https://apps.who.int/iris/bitstream/handle/10665/43894/97892?sequence=1.
86. G. Alcelik et al., "Treatment of Iron Deficiency Anemia Induces Weight Loss and Improves Metabolic Parameters," La Clinica Terapeutica 165, no. 2 (2014): 87-89, doi: 10.7471/CT.2014.1688.
87. Gulsum Emel Pamuk et al., "Gastrointestinal Symptoms Are Closely Associated with Depression in Iron Deficiency Anemia: A Comparative Study," ASM Annals of Saudi Medicine 35, no. 1 (2015), https://doi.org/10.5144/0256-4947.2015.31.
88. "Ferritin Test," Mayo Clinic online, December 28, 2021, https://www.mayoclinic.org/tests-procedures/ferritin-test/about/pac-20384928.

89   Rajiv Heda, Fadi Toro, and Claudio R. Tombazzi, "Physiology, Pepsin," last modified May 8, 2022, https://www.ncbi.nlm.nih.gov/books/NBK537005/.

90   Anne Thiel, "The Role of Hydrochloric Acid (Hcl) in Aiding Digestion," last modified December 3, 2019, https://www. integrativepro.com/articles/the-role-of-hydrochloric-acid-in-aiding-digestion.

91   Maria Fischer, "How Much Protein Can Your Body Absorb?" Gainful online, last modified October 14, 2020, https://www.gainful.com/blog/how-much-protein-can-your-body-absorb/.

92   Jamie I. Baum, Il-Young Kim, Robert R. Wolfe, "Protein Consumption and the Elderly: What Is the Optimal Level of Intake?" Nutrients 8, no. 6 (2016): 359, doi: 10.3390/nu8060359.

93   Ji Hyun, Se Ryung, and Jong Seung Kim, "Relationship between Low Muscle Mass and Metabolic Syndrome in Elderly People with Normal Body Mass Index," Journal of Bone Metabolism 22, no, 3 (2015): 99-106, doi: 10.11005/jbm.2015.22.3.99.

94   Kenta Yamamoto et al., "Patients with Low Muscle Mass Have Characteristic Microbiome with Low Potential for Amino Acid Synthesis in Chronic Liver Disease," Scientific Reports 12, 3674 (2022), doi: 10.1038/s41598-022-07810-3.

95   Nicolaas E. P. Deutz et al., "The Underappreciated Role of Low Muscle Mass in the Management of Malnutrition," Journal of American Medical Directors Association 20, no. 1 (2019), https//doi.org/doi: 10.1016/j.jamda.2018.11.01.

96   "Probiotics," Cleveland Clinic online, last modified March 9, 2020, https://my.clevelandclinic.org/health/articles/14598-probiotics.

97   Emily Nock, "What are Polyphenols? Another Great Reason to Eat Fruits and Veggies," last modified June 2021, https://www.chhs.colostate.edu/krnc/monthly-blog/what-are-polyphenols-another-great-reason-to-eat-fruits-and-veggies/.

98   M. Feldman et al., "Effects of Aging and Gastritis on Gastric Acid and Pepsin Secretion in Humans: A Prospective Study," Gastroenterology 110, no. 4 (1996): 1043-1052, doi: 10.1053/gast.1996.v110.pm8612992.

99   "Sarcopenia," Cleveland Clinic online, last modified June 3, 2022, https://my.clevelandclinic.org/health/diseases/23167-sarcopenia.

100 "Iron Deficiency Anemia," Mayo Clinic online, accessed April 4, 2023, https://www.mayoclinic.org/diseases-conditions/iron-deficiency-anemia/symptoms-causes/syc-20355034.

101 "Vitamin B12," Harvard T.H. Chan School of Public Health online, last modified March 2023, https://www.hsph.harvard.edu/nutritionsource/vitamin-b12/.

102 "The Unusual Link Between Low Stomach Acid and Osteoporosis," University Health News Daily online, May 5, 2020, https://universityhealthnews.com/daily/bones-joints/osteoporosis-could-low-stomach-acid-be-the-cause-of-your-bone-health-problems/.

103 Noah Ghossein, Michael Kang, and Anand D. Lakhar, "Anticholinergic Medications," last modified May 16, 2022, https://www.ncbi.nlm.nih.gov/books/NBK555893/.

104 Raymond F. Orzechowski, Debra S. Currie, and Cathryn A. Valancius, "Comparative Anticholinergic Activities of 10 Histamine H1 Receptor Antagonists in Two Functional Models," European Journal of Pharmacology 506, no.. 3 (2004): 257-264, doi: 10.1016/j.ejphar.2004.11.006.

105 A. Garner, H. Fadlallah, and M.E. Parsons, "1976 and all that! - 20 years of antisecretory therapy," Gut 39, no. 6 (1996): 784-786, doi: 10.1136/gut.39.6.784.

106 Ichoro Yoshikawa et al., "Long-term Treatment with Proton Pump Inhibitor is Associated with Undesired Weight Gain," World Journal of Gastroenterology 15, no. 38 (2009): 4794-4798, doi: 10.3748/wjg.15.4794.

107 "Omeprazole: Drug Usage Statistics, United States, 2013 – 2020," Clincalc.com, accessed on April 1, 2023. https://clincalc.com/DrugStats/Drugs/Omeprazole

108 Blake H. Salisbury and Jamie M. Terrell, "Antiacids," last modified August 15, 2022, https://www.ncbi.nlm.nih.gov/books/NBK526049/.

109 "Acid Reflux (GER & GERD) in Adults," National Institute of Diabetes and Digestive and Kidney Diseases, accessed April 4, 2023, https://www.niddk.nih.gov/health-information/digestive-diseases/acid-reflux-ger-gerd-adults.

110 John V. Fahy and Burton F. Dickey, "Airway Mucus Function and Dysfunction," New England Journal of Medicine 323, no. 23 (2010): 2233-2247, doi: 10.1056/NEJMra0910061.

111 "Proton Pump Inhibitors," MedlinePlus online, last modified April 22, 2021, https://medlineplus.gov/ency/patientinstructions/000381.htm.

112 Andrew Bennett Hellman, "Gut Bacteria Gene Complement Dwarfs Human Genome," last modified March 3, 2010, https://doi.org/10.1038/news.2010.104.

113 Baohong Wang et al., "The Human Microbiota in Health and Disease," Engineering 3, no. 1 (2017): 71-82, https://doi.org/10.1016/J ENG.2017.01.008.

114 "Humans are Made up of More Microbes than Human Cells," Wired online, June 15, 2012, https://www.wired.co.uk/article/human-microbes.

115 Xing Yang et al, "More than 9,000,000 Unique Genes in Human Gut Bacterial Community: Estimating Gene Numbers Inside a Human Body," PLoS One 4, no. 6 (June 2009). https://www.ncbi.nlm.nih.gov/pmc/articles/PMC2699651/

116 Christopher D. Link, "Is There a Brain Microbiome?" Sage Journals online, accessed April 4, 2023, https://journals.sagepub.com/doi/full/10.1177/26331055211018709.

117 Ibid.

118 Carrie A.M. Wegh et al., "Postbiotics and Their Potential Applications in Early Life Nutrition and Beyond," International Journal of Molecular Sciences 20, no. 19 (2019): 4673, doi:10.3390/ijms20194673.

119 Glenn R. Gibson et al., "Expert Consensus Document: The International Scientific Association for Probiotics and Prebiotics (ISAPP) Consensus Statement on the Definition and Scope of Prebiotics," Nature Reviews Gastroenterology & Hepatology 14 (2017): 491-502, doi: https://doi.org/10.1038/nrgastro.2017.75.

120 John Wallace and Dwight Lingenfelter, "Glyphosate (Roundup): Understanding Risks to Human Health," last modfied January 5, 2023, https://extension.psu.edu/glyphosate-roundup-understanding-risks-to-human-health.

121 Jose V. Tarazona et al., "Glyphosate Toxicity and Carcinogenicity: A review of the Scientific Basis of the European Union Assessment and its Differences with IARC," Archives of Toxicology 91 (2017): 2723-2743, doi: https://doi.org/10.1007/s00204-017-1962-5.

122 Malcom Weir, "Applying Ointment, Creams, and Lotions on Dogs," last April 4, 2023, https://vcahospitals.com/know-your-pet/applying-ointments-creams-and-lotions-on-dogs.

123 Amy Langdon, Nathan Crook, and Gautam Dantas, "The effects of Antibiotics on the Microbiome Throughout Development and Alternative Approaches for Therapeutic Modulation," Genome Medicine 8, no. 39 (2016), doi: https://doi.org/10.1186/s13073-016-0294-z.

124 Olli Turta and Samuli Rautava, "Antibiotics, Obesity and the Link to Microbes - What are We doing to Our Children?" BMC Medicine 14, no. 57 (2016), doi: https://doi.org/10.1186/s12916-016-0605-7.

125 Karen S. W. Leong et al., "Antibiotics, Gut Microbiome and Obesity," Clin Endocrinol (Oxf) 88, no. 2 (2017): 185-200, doi: 10.1111/cen.13495.

126 Cecila Jernberg et al., "Long-term Impacts of Antibiotic Exposure on the Human Intestinal Microbiota," PubMed 156, no. 11 (2010): 3216-3223, doi: 10.1099/mic.0.040618-0.

127 Howard F. Loomis, "Digestion in the Stomach," accessed April 4, 2023, https://www.foodenzymeinstitute.com/content/Digestion-in-the-Stomach.aspx.

128 Deepshika Ramaan and Ken Cadwell, "Intrinsic Defense Mechanisms of the Intestinal Epithelium," Cell Host Microbe 19, no. 4 (2017): 434-441, doi: 10.1016/j.chom.2016.03.003.

129 Ibid.

130 James M. Anderson and Christina M. Van Itallie, "Physiology and Functions of Tight Junctions," Cold Spring Harbor Perspectives in Biology 1, no. 2 (2009), a002585, doi: 10.1101/cshperspect.a002584.

131 Takuya Suzuki, "Regulation of the Intestinal Barrier by Nutrients: The Role of Tight Junctions," Animal Science Journal 92, no. 1 (2020): e13357, doi: 10.1111/asj.13357.

132 "Leaky Gut Syndrome," Cleveland Clinic online, last modified April 6, 2022, https://my.clevelandclinic.org/health/diseases/22724-leaky-gut-syndrome.

133 Marcelo Campos, "Leaky Gut: What Is It, and What Does it Mean for You?" last modified November 16, 2021, https://www.health.harvard.edu/blog/leaky-gut-what-is-it-and-what- does-it-mean-for-you-2017092212451.

134 Vanuytsel, T., S. Vermeire, and I. Cleynen. "The role of Haptoglobin and its related protein, Zonulin, in inflammatory bowel disease," Tissue Barriers 1, no. 5 (2013):e27321. doi: 10.4161/tisb.27321. Epub 2013 Dec 10. PMID: 24868498; PMCID: PMC3943850.

135 Alessio Fasana, "Regulation of Tight Junctions, and Autoimmune Diseases," Annals of the New York Academy of Sciences 1258, no. 1 (2012): 25-33, doi: 10.1111/j.1749-6632. 2012.06538.x.

136 Michael F. Cusik, Jane E. Libbey, and Robert S. Fujinami, "Molecular Mimicry as a Mechanism of Autoimmune Disease," Clinical Reviews in Allergy and Immunology 42, no. 1 (2011): 102-111, doi: 10.1007/s12016-011-8294-7.

137 "Hashimoto's Thyroiditis," Johns Hopkins Medicine, accessed April 4, 2023, https://www.hopkinsmedicine.org/health/conditions-and-diseases/hashimotos-thyroiditis.

138 Monika Ostrowska et al., "Cartilage and Bone Damage in Rheumatoid Arthritis," Reumatologia 52, no. 2 (2018): 111-120, doi: 10.5114/reum.2018.75523.

139 Katya Orlova, "How Does Diabetes Increase Risk for Pancreatitis?" Ariel Precision Medicine, April 27, 2020, https://arielmedicine.com/how-does-diabetes-increase-risk-for-pancreatitis/.

140 Jessica Lau, "Epidemic of Autoimmune Diseases Calls for Action," last modified January 31, 2019, https://news.harvard.edu/gazette/story/2019/01/epidemic-of-autoimmune-diseases -pushes-researchers-in-new-direction/

141 Qinghui Mu et al., "Leaky Gut as a Danger Signal for Autoimmune Diseases," Frontiers in Immunology 8 (2017), https://doi.org/ 10.3389/fimmu.2017.00598.

142 Rima M. Chakaroun, Lucas Massier, and Peter Kovacs, "Gut Microbiome, Intestinal Permeability, and Tissue Bacteria in Metabolic Disease: Perpetrators or Bystanders?" Nutrients 12, no. 4 (2020): 1082, doi: 10.3390/nu12041982.

143 Ravinder Nagpal et al., "Obesity-Linked Gut Microbiome Dysbiosis Associated with Derangements in Gut Permeability and Intestinal Cellular," J Diabetes Res (2018), doi: 10.1155/2018/3462092.

144 Paul Trayhurn, "Oxygen—A Critical, but Overlooked, Nutrient," Frontiers in Nutrition 6, no 1 (2019), doi; https://doi.org/10.3389%2Ffnut.2019.00010.

145 Luc Staner, "Sleep and Anxiety Disorders," Dialogues of in Clinical Neuroscience 5, no. 3 (2003): 249-258, doi; 10.31887/DCNS.2003.5.3/lstaner.

146 "Hypoxemia," last modified March 24, 2023, https://www.mayoclinic.org/symptoms/hypoxemia/basics/causes/sym-20050930.

147 Bruce Ames and Rhonda Patrick, "Bruce Ames on Triage Theory, Longevity Vitamins & Micronutrients," Found My Fitness, February 15, 2015, video, 46:58, https://www.foundmyfitness.com/episodes/bruce-ames.

148 Joyce C. McCann and Bruce N. Ames, "Vitamin K, an Example of Triage Theory: Is Micronutrient Inadequacy Linked to Diseases of Aging?" The American Journal of Clinical Nutrition 90, no. 4 (2009): 889-907, doi: 10.3945/ajcn.2009.27930.

149 "Vitamin K," Harvard T.H. Chan School of Public Health online, last modified March 2023, https://www.hsph.harvard.edu/nutritionsource/vitamin-k/.

150 "Methylmalonic Acid (MMA) Test," Mediline Plus online, November 16, 2021, https://medlineplus.gov/lab-tests/methylmalonic-acid-mma-test/.

151 "Stages of Nutrient Deficiency," Chegg, accessed April 4, 2023, https://www.chegg.com/learn/topic/stages-of-deficiency-nutrient.

152 Garland, S.N., H. Rowe, L.M. Repa, K. Fowler, E.S. Zhou, and M.A. Grandner, "A decade's difference: 10-year change in insomnia symptom prevalence in Canada depends on sociodemographics and health status," Sleep Health 4, no. 2 (2018): 160-165, doi: 10.1016/j.sleh.2018.01.003. Epub 2018 Feb 19. PMID: 29555129; PMCID: PMC6203592.

153 Galland-Decker, C., P. Marques-Vidal, and P. Vollenweider, "Prevalence and factors associated with fatigue in the Lausanne middle-aged population: a population-based, cross-sectional survey," BMJ Open 9, no. 8 (2019):e027070. doi: 10.1136/bmjopen-2018-027070. PMID: 31446404; PMCID: PMC6720133.

154 "Scientific Report of the 2015 Dietary Guidelines Advisory Committee," Secretary of Health and Human Services and the Secretary of Agriculture, accessed April 5, 2023, https://health.gov/sites/default/files/2019-09/Scientific-Report-of-the-2015-Dietary-Guidelines-Advisory-Committee.pdf.

155 "Top 250: The Ranking," Restaurant Business, accessed April 5, 2023, https://www.restaurantbusinessonline.com/top-500-chains?year=2021&page=0#data-table.

156 Neelima Panth et al., "The Influence of Diet on Fertility and the Implications for Public Health Nutrition in the United States," Front Public Health 6, no. 211 (2018): 211, doi: 10.3389/fpubh.2018.00211.

157 "Scientific Report of the 2015 Dietary Guidelines Advisory Committee," Secretary of Health and Human Services and the Secretary of Agriculture, accessed April 5, 2023, https://health.gov/sites/default/files/2019-09/Scientific-Report-of-the-2015-Dietary-Guidelines-Advisory-Committee.pdf.

158 Lisa Russell, "Processed vs. Unprocessed Foods: Getting the Facts," last modified September 7, 2021, https://www.midriversnewsmagazine.com/online_features/health_and_wellness/processed-vs-unprocessed-foods-getting-the-facts/article_884b6f6f-9167-5441-885d-afce759cd042.html.

159 Lovely Gupta et al., "The Twin White Herrings: Salt and Sugar," Indian Journal of Endocrinology and Metabolism 22, no. 4 (2018): 542-551, doi; 10.4103/ijem.IJEM_117_18.

160 Carlos Augusto Monteiro et al., Ultra-processed Foods, Diet Quality, and Health Using the NOVA Classification System, (Food and Agriculture Organization of the United Nations, 2019), https://www.fao.org/3/ca5644en/ca5644en.pdf.

161 Anaïs Rico-Campà et al., "Association Between Consumption of Ultra-Processed Foods and All Cause Mortality: SUN Prospective Cohort Study," BMJ 365 (2019), doi: 10.1136/bmj.l1949.

162 Bernard Srour et al., "Ultra-Processed Food Intake and Risk of Cardiovascular Disease: Prospective Cohort Study (NutriNet-Santé)," BMJ 365 (2019), doi: 10.1136/bmj.l1451.Srour B, Fezeu L K, Kesse-Guyot E, AllÃ¨s B, MÃ©jean C, Andrianasolo R M et al., Ultra-processed food intake and risk of cardiovascular disease: prospective cohort study (NutriNet-Santé) BMJ 2019; 365 :l1451 doi:10.1136/bmj.l1451

163 Anaïs Rico-Campà et al., "Association Between Consumption of Ultra-Processed Foods and All Cause Mortality: SUN Prospective Cohort Study," BMJ 365 (2019), doi: 10.1136/bmj.l1949.

164 Hayami K. Koga et al., "Optimism, Lifestyle, and Longevity in a Racially Diverse Cohort of Women," Journal of the American Geriatrics Society 70, no. 10 (2022): 2793-2804, doi; 10.1111/jgs.17897.

165 Linda G. Russek and Gary E. Schwartz, "Feeling of Parental Caring Predict Health Status in Midlife: A 35-Year Follow-up of the Harvard Mastery of Stress Study," Journal of Behavioral Medicine 20 (1997): 1-13, doi: 10.1023/A:1025525428213.

166 Vincent J. Felitti, "The Between Adverse Childhood Experiences and Adult Health: Turning Gold into Lead," The Permanente Journal 6, no. 1 (2002): 44-47, doi: 10.7812/tpp/02.994.

167 Lisanne M.M. Gommers et al., "Hypomagnesemia in Type 2 Diabetes: A Vicious Circle?" Diabetes 1 (2016): 3-13, doi: 10.2337/db15-1028.

168 Abigail May Khan et al., "Low Serum Magnesium and the Development of Atrial Fibrillation in the Community," Circulation 127, 1 (2013): 2-4, doi: 10.1161/CIR.0b013e31828293c1.

169 "Take the ACE Quiz – And Learn What It Does and Doesn't Mean," Harvard University Center on the Developing Child, accessed April 5, 2023, https://developingchild.harvard.edu/media-coverage/take-the-ace-quiz-and-learn-what-it-does-and-doesnt-mean/.

170 Emily S. Mohn et al., "Evidence of Drug-Nutrient Interactions with Chronic Use of Commonly Prescribed Medications: An Update," Pharmaceutics 10, no. 1 (2018): 36, doi: 10.3390/pharmaceutics10010036.

171 Richard Deichmann, Carl Lavie, and Samuel Andrews, "Coenzyme Q10 and Statin-Induced Mitochondrial Dysfunction," The Ochsner Journal 10, no. 1 (2010): 16-21, doi: 10.1136/bmj.l1580.

172 Yan Xie et al., "Estimates of All Cause Mortality and Cause Specific Mortality Associated with Proton Pump Inhibitors Among US Veterans: Cohort Study," BMJ 365 (2019), doi: 10.1136/bmj.11580.

173 Hastuti Tajuddin et al., "Insulin Therapy Increases the Risk of Hypokalemia and Arrhythmia in Diabetic Patients with Coronary Heart Disease: A Retrospective Study in Wahidin Sudirohusodo General Hospital," Galenkika Journal of Pharmacy (e-Journal) 8, no. 2 (2002), doi: 10.22487/j24428744.2022.v8.i2.15930.

174 W.P. Leary and A.J. Reyes, "Diuretic-Induced Magnesium Losses," Drugs 28 (1984): 182-187, doi: 10.2165/00003495-198400281-00018.

175 Maura Palmery et al., "Oral Contraceptives and Changes in Nutritional Requirements," European Review for Medical Pharmacological Sciences 17, no. 13 (2013): 1804-1813, PMID: 23852908.

176 Neil Vargesson, "Thalidomide-Induced Teratogenesis: History and Mechanisms," Birth Defects Research 105 (2015): 140-156, doi: 10.1002/bdrc.21096.

177 Lina Felípez and Timothy A. Sentongo, "Drug-Induced Nutrient Deficiencies," Pediatric Clinics of North America 56, no. 5 (2009): 1211-1224, doi; 10.1016/j.plc.2009.06.004.

178 Igho J. Onakpoya, Carl J. Heneghan, and Jeffrey K. Aronson, "Post-Marketing Withdrawal of 462 Medicinal Products Because of Adverse Drug Reactions: A Systematic Review of the World Literature," BMC Medicine 14, no. 10 (2016, corrected 2019), doi: 10.1186/s12916-016-0553-2.

179 Dennis Miller, "Why Aren't Pharmacists Critical of Pharmaceuticals?" last modified January 12, 2021, https://www.peoplespharmacy.com/articles/why-arent-pharmacists-critical-of-pharmaceuticals.

180 "Heat, medications don't mix," Baylor College of Medicine, accessed on April 1, 2023. https://www.bcm.edu/news/heat-medications-dont-mix.

181 Sophie M.T. Wehrens et al., "Meal Timing Regulates the Human Circadian System," Current Biology 27, no. 12 (2017): 1768-1775.eb, doi: 10.1016/j.cub.2017.04.059.

182 Roberto Buono and Valter D. Longo, "When Fasting Gets Tough, the Tough Immune Cells Get Going-or Die," Cell 178, no. 5 (2019): 1038-1040, doi: 10.1016/j.cell.2019.07.052.

183 Noboro Mizushimi et al., "Autophagy Fights Disease Through Cellular Self-Digestion," Nature 451, no. 7181 (2017): 1069-1075, doi: 10.1038/nature06639.

184 Bret H. Goodpaster and Lauren M. Sparks, "Metabolic Flexibility in Health and Disease," Cell Metabolism 25, no. 5 (2017): 1027-1036, doi: 10.1016/j.cmet.2017.04.015.

185 Rong Hou et al., "Cold and Hungry: Combined Effects of Low Temperature and Resource Scarcity on an Edge-of-Range Temperate primate, the Golden Snub-Nose Monkey," Ecography 43, no. 11 (2020): 1672-1682, doi: 10.1111/ecog.05295.

186 Richard J. Johnson et al., "Perspective: A Historical and Scientific Perspective of Sugar and Its Relation with Obesity and Diabetes," Advances in Nutrition 8, p. 3 (2017): 412-422, doi: doi:10.3945/an.116.014654.

187 Jon Johnson, "What's to Know About Insulin Overdose?" last modified April 14, 2019, https://www.medicalnewstoday.com/articles/317300#symptoms.

188 Saidur Rahman et al., "Role of Insulin in Health and Disease: An Update," International Journal of Molecular Sciences 22, no.12 (2021): 6403, doi: 10.3390/ijms22126403.

189 "The Liver & Blood Sugar," Diabetes Education Online, accessed April 5, 2023, https://dtc.ucsf.edu/types-of-diabetes/type1/understanding-type-1-diabetes/how-the-body-processes-sugar/the-liver-blood-sugar/.

190 "Glyburide," MedlinePlus online, last modified October 15, 2018, https://medlineplus.gov/druginfo/meds/a684058.html.

191 Angela M. Bell, "How Insulin and Glucagon Regulate Blood Sugar," last modified September 12, 2022, https://www.medicalnewstoday.com/articles/316427.

192 Gugliucci Alejandro, "Formation of Fructose-Mediated Advanced Glycation End Products and Their Roles in Metabolic and Inflammatory Diseases," Advances in Nutrition 8, no. 1 (2017): 54-62, doi: 10.3945/an.116.013912.

[193] Chan-Sik Kim, Sok Park, and Junghyun Kim, "The Role of Glycation in the Pathogenesis of Aging and its Prevention Through Herbal Products and Physical Exercise," Journal of Exercise Nutrition & Biochemistry 21, no. 3 (2017): 55-61, doi: 10.20463/jenb.2017.0027.

[194] Filipa C. Simões and Paul R. Riley, "Immune Cells in Cardiac Repair and Regeneration," Development 149, no. 8 (2022): dev199906, doi: 10.1242/dev.199906.

[195] Anastasia Poznyak et al., "The Diabetes Mellitus–Atherosclerosis Connection: The Role of Lipid and Glucose Metabolism and Chronic Inflammation," International Journal of Molecular Sciences 21, no. 5 (2020): 1835, doi: .10.3390/ijms21051835.

[196] W. Todd Cade, "Diabetes-Related Microvascular and Macrovascular Diseases in the Physical Therapy Setting," Physical Therapy 88, no. 11 (2008): 1322-1335, doi: .10.2522/ptj.20080008.

[197] Raffaele Pallandino et al., "Association Between Pre-Diabetes and Microvascular and Macrovascular Disease in Newly Diagnosed Type 2 Diabetes," BMJ Open Diabetes Open Research & Care 8. No. 1 (2020): e001061, doi: 10.1136/bmjdrc-2019-001061.

[198] Suzanne M. de la Monte, "Alzheimer's Disease is Type 3 Diabetes-Evidence Reviewed," Journal of Diabetes Science and Technology 2, no. 6 (2008): 1101-1113, doi: 10.1177/193229680800200619.

[199] Adam G. Tabák et al., "Prediabetes: A High-Risk State for Diabetes Development," Lancet 379, no. 9833 (2012): 2279-2290, doi: 10.1016/s0140-6736(12)60283-9.

[200] "Blood Sugar (Sugar) Test," Cleveland Clinic online, last modified November 16, 2022, https://my.clevelandclinic.org/health/diagnostics/12363-blood-glucose-test.

[201] https://www.levelshealth.com/blog/what-should-my-glucose-levels-be-ultimate-guide.

[202] Dylan D. Thomas et al., "Hyperinsulinemia: An Early Indicator of Metabolic Dysfunction," Journal of Endocrine System 3, no. 9 (2019): 1727-1747, doi: .10.1210/js.2019-00065.

203 Frank B. Hu et al., "Elevated Risk of Cardiovascular Disease Prior to Clinical Diagnosis of Type 2 Diabetes," Diabetes Care 25, no. 7 (2002): 1129-1134, doi: 10.2337/diacare.25.7.1129.

204 Michael F. Jacobson, "Buying the Snackwell Myth," last modified December 11, 2015, https://medium.com/@CSPI/burying-the-snackwell-myth-4b6e9dff6d07.

205 John S. White, "Straight Talk About High-Fructose Corn Syrup: What It Is and What It Ain't," The American Journal of Clinical Nutrition 88, no. 6 (2008): 1716S-1721S, doi: 10.3945/ajcn.2008.25825B.

206 M. Yanin Pepino, "Metabolic Effects of Non-Nutritive Sweeteners," Physiology & Behavior 152, no. 0 0 (2015): 450-455, doi: 10.1016/j.physbeh.2015.06.024rehend.

207 Marie M.S. Palmnäs et al., "Low-Dose Aspartame Consumption Differentially Affects Gut Microbiota-Host Metabolic Interactions in the Diet-Induced Obese Rat," PLoS One 9, no. 10 (2014): e109841, doi: 10.1371/journal.pone.0109841.

208 Mary V. Burke and Dana M. Small, "Physiological Mechanisms by Which Non-Nutritive Sweeteners May Impact Body Weight and Metabolism," Physiology & Behavior 152, no. Pt B (2015): 381-388, doi: 10.1016/j.physbeh.2015.05.036.

209 Alexandra G. Yunker et al., "Obesity and Sex-Related Associations with Differential Effects of Sucralose vs Sucrose on Appetite and Reward Processing: A Randomized Crossover Trial," JAMA Network Open 4, no. 9 (2021): e2126313, doi: 10.1001/jamanetworkopen.2021.26313.

210 "Carbohydrates and Blood Sugar," Harvard T.H. Chan School of Public Health, accessed April 5, 2023, https://www.hsph.harvard.edu/nutritionsource/carbohydrates/carbohydrates-and-blood-sugar/.

211 Gabriele Riccardi and Angela Rivellese, "Effects of Dietary Fiber and Carbohydrate on Glucose Diabetes Care," Diabetes Care 14, no. 12 (1991): 1115-1125, doi: 10.2337/diacare.14.12.1115.

212 Yunshang Ma et al., "Association Between Dietary Fiber and Markers of Systemic Inflammation in the Women's Health Initiative Observational Study," Nutrition 24, no. 10 (2008): 941-949, doi: 10.1016/j.nut.2008.04.005.

[213] Alison B. Evert et al., "Nutrition Therapy for Adults with Diabetes or Prediabetes: A Consensus Report," Diabetes Care 42, no. 5 (2019): 731-754, doi: .10.2337/dci19-0014.

[214] Dan Buettner and Sam Skemp, "Blue Zones: Lessons from the World's Longest Lived," American Journal of Lifestyle Medicine 10, no. 5 (2016): 318-321, doi: 10.1177/1559827616637066; Dagfinn Aune et al., "Whole Grain Consumption and Risk of Cardiovascular Disease, Cancer, and all Cause and Cause Specific Mortality: Systematic Review and Dose-Response Meta-Analysis of Prospective Studies," BJM 353 (2016), doi: 10.1136/bmj.i2716.

[215] Bret H. Goodpaster and Lauren M. Sparks, "Metabolic Flexibility in Health and Disease," Cell Metabolism 25, no. 5 (2017): 1027-1036, doi: 10.1016/j.cmet.2017.04.015.

[216] Kerri-Ann Jennings, "16 Easy Ways to Eat More Fiber," last modified February 14, 2023, https://www.healthline.com/nutrition/16-ways-to-eat-more-fiber.

[217] "Water," LibreTexts online, last modified November 15, 2021, https://bio.libretexts.org/Bookshelves/Introductory_and_General_Biology/Book%3A_Principles_of_Biology/01%3A_Chapter_1/02%3A_Chemistry_for_Biology/2.03%3A_Water.

[218] Jane Higdon, "Sodium (Chloride)," last modified April 11, 2019, https://lpi.oregonstate.edu/mic/minerals/sodium#LPI-recommendation.

[219] Ozgur C. Eren et al., "Multilayered Interplay Between Fructose and Salt in Development of Hypertension," Hypertension 73, no. 2 (2019): 265-272, doi: .10.1161/HYPERTENSIONAHA.118.12150.

[220] "The Effects: Human Health," United States Environmental Protection Agency, last modified March 30, 2023, https://www.epa.gov/nutrientpollution/effects-human-health.

[221] Perry Zeitz Ruckart et al., "The Flint Water Crisis: A Coordinated Public Health Emergency Response and Recovery Initiative," J Public Health Manag Pract. (2019): S84-S90, doi: 10.1097/PHH.0000000000000871.

222 Lucy Shouten, "Most Americans Don't Drink (or Trust) Tap Water: Should They?" last modified March 5, 2016, https://www.csmonitor.com/Environment/2016/0305/Most-Americans-don-t-drink-or-trust-tap-water-Should-they.

223 Michael Phillis, "US Pushes for Better Tap Water but Must Win Over Wary Public," last modified January 30, 2022, https://apnews.com/article/environment-and-nature-michigan-water-quality-flint-b843f813feea5eddd43d10181204b054; Asher Rosinger, "Nearly 60 Million Americans Don't Drink Their Tap Water, Research Suggests – Here's Why That's a Public Health Problem," accessed April 5, 2023, https://theconversation.com/nearly-60-million-americans-dont-drink-their-tap-water-research-suggests-heres-why-thats-a-public-health-problem-158483.

224 Daichi Nakamura et al., "Bisphenol A May Cause Testosterone Reduction by Adversely Affecting Both Testis and Pituitary Systems Similar to Estradiol," Toxicology Letters 194, no. 1-2 (2010): 16-25, doi: 10.1016/j.toxlet.2010.02.002.

225 Joe M. Braun, "Bisphenol A and Children's Health," Curr Opin Pediatr 23, no. 2 (2011): 233-239, doi: 10.1097/MOP.0b013e3283445675.

226 Xiaoqian Gao and Hong-Sheng Wang, "Impact of Bisphenol A on the Cardiovascular System — Epidemiological and Experimental Evidence and Molecular Mechanisms," Int. J. Environ. Res. Public Health 11, no. 8 (2014): 8399-8413, doi: 10.3390/ijerph110808399.

227 Michele La Merrill et al., "Toxicological Function of Adipose Tissue: Focus on Persistent Organic Pollutants," Environ Health Perspect 121, no. 2 (2013): 162-169, doi; 10.1289/ehp.1205485.

228 Bruce Blumberg and Raquel Chamorro-Garicia, "Is Plastic Making Us Fat?" last modified August 23, 2018, https://www.universityofcalifornia.edu/news/are-we-gaining-weight-plastic.

229 "Project 1: Superfund Chemicals, Nutrition, and Multi-Organ Cardiovascular Risk," Superfund Research Center, accessed April 5, 2023, https://superfund.engr.uky.edu/project-1.

230 Barry M. Popkin, Kristen E. D'Anci, and Irwin H. Rosenberg, "Water, Hydration, and Health," Nutr Nev 68, no. 8 (2010): 439-458, 10.1111/j.1753-4887.2010.00304.x.

231 R.A. DeFronzo et al., "The Effect of Insulin on Renal Handling of Sodium, Potassium, Calcium, and Phosphate in Man," J Clin Invest. 55, no. 4 (1975): 845-855, doi: .10.1172/JCI107996.

232 "History and Timeline of Soft Drinks," History of Soft Drinks, last accessed April 5, 2023, http://www.historyofsoftdrinks.com/soft-drink-history/timeline-of-soft-drinks/.

233 https://www.dietaryguidelines.gov/sites/default/files/2020-12/Dietary_Guidelines_for_Americans_2020-2025.pdf#page=31.

234 R.J. Maughan and J. Griffin, "Caffeine Ingestion and Fluid Balance: A Review," J Hum Nutr Diet. 16, no. 6 (2003): 411-420, doi: 10.1046/j.1365-277x.2003.00477.x.

235 Vasani S. Malik and Mattias B. Schulze, "Intake of Sugar-Sweetened Beverages and Weight Gain: A Systematic Review," Am J Clin Nutr 84, no. 2 (2006): doi:10.1093/ajcn/84.1.274; William Nseir, Fares Nassar, and Nimer Assy, "Soft Drinks Consumption and Nonalcoholic Fatty Liver Disease," World J Gastronenterol 16, no. 21 (2010); 2579-2588, doi: doi:10.3748/wjg.v16.i21.2579.

236 Amy Mullee et al., "Association Between Soft Drink Consumption and Mortality in 10 European Countries," JAMA Intern Med. 179, no. 11 (2019): 1479-1490, doi: 10.1001/jamainternmed.2019.2478.

237 Babak Mokhlesi et al., "Evaluation and Management of Obesity Hypoventilation Syndrome. An Official American Thoracic Society Clinical Practice Guideline," Am J Respir Crit Care Med 200, no. 3 (2019): e6-e24, doi: 10.1164/rccm.201905-1071ST.

238 Maxx P. Horowitz and J. Timothy Greenamyre, "Mitochondrial Iron Metabolism and its Role in Neurodegeneration," J Alzheimers Dis 20 Suppl 2, Suppl 2 (2010): S551-S568, doi:10.3233/JAD-2010-100354; Bibbin T. Paul et al., "Mitochondria and Iron: Current Questions," Expert Rev Hematal 10, no. 1 (2016): 65-79, doi: 10.1080/17474086.2016.1268047.

239 "Micronutrients," World Health Organization, accessed April 5, 2023, https://www.who.int/health-topics/micronutrients#tab=tab_1.

240 Esa T. Soppi, "Iron Deficiency Without Anemia – A Clinical Challenge," Clinical Case Reports 6, no. 6 (2018): 1082-1086, doi: 10.1002/ccr3.1529.

241 "Iron-Deficiency Anemia," American Society of Hematology, accessed April 6, 2023, https://www.hematology.org/education/patients/anemia/iron-deficiency.

242 "10 Interesting Things About Air," NASA online, last modified September 12, 2016, https://climate.nasa.gov/news/2491/10-interesting-things-about-air/.

243 "Particle Pollution," CDC online, last modified February 16, 2023, https://www.cdc.gov/air/particulate_matter.html.

244 "Air Pollution," CDC online, last modified December 21, 2020, https://www.cdc.gov/climateandhealth/effects/air_pollution.htm.

245 Air Pollution Linked to Dementia Cases," National Institutes of Health, September 5, 2023, https://www.nih.gov/news-events/nih-research-matters/air-pollution-linked-dementia-cases.

246 "Air Pollution and Your Health," National Institute of Environmental Health Sciences, accessed April 6, 2023, https://www.niehs.nih.gov/health/topics/agents/air-pollution/index.cfm.

247 "Learning Diaphragmatic Breathing," Harvard Health Publishing, Harvard Medical School, last modified March 10, 2016, https://www.health.harvard.edu/healthbeat/learning-diaphragmatic-breathing.

248 Ana Gotter, "Breathing Exercises to Increase Lung Capacity," last modified September 29, 2022, https://www.healthline.com/health/how-to-increase-lung-capacity.

249 "Fitness Market Size, Revenue & Growth 2023 [+ Research Report]," Wellness Creative Co., accessed April 6, 2023, https://www.wellnesscreatives.com/fitness-market/.

250 H. Pontzer, B.M. Wood, and D.A. Raichler, "Hunter-Gathers as Models in Public Health," Obes Rev 19, Suppl 1 (2018): doi: 10.1111/obr.12785.

251 Dan Buettner and Sam Skemp, "Blue Zones: Lessons from the World's Longest Lived," Am J Lifestyle Med 10, no. 5 (2016): 5045-5046, doi: 10.1177/1559827616637066.

252 Darren P. Casey and Emma C. Hart, "Cardiovascular Function in Humans During Exercise: Role of the Muscle Pump," J Physiol 586, no. 21 (2008): 5045-5046, doi: 10.1113/jphysiol.2008.162123.

253 "Balance and Aging," Vestibular Disorders Association, accessed April 6, 2023, https://www.networks.nhs.uk/nhs-networks/tai-chi-for-health-and-rehabilitation-london-uk/documents/file.2019-06-10.5134964040.

254 Valter Santilli et al., "Clinical Definition of Sarcopenia," Clin Cases Miner Bone Metab 11, no. 3 (2014): 177-180, PMCID: PMC4269139, PMID: 25568649.

255 Evelyn Ferri et al., "Role of Age-Related Mitochondrial Dysfunction in Sarcopenia," Int J Mol Sci. 21, no. 15 (2020): 5236, doi: 10.3390/ijms21155236.

256 Sung-Young Jang et al., "Low Muscle Mass is Associated with Osteoporosis: A Nationwide Population-Based Study," Maturitas March, no. 133 (2020): 54-59, doi: 10.1016/j.maturitas.2020.01.003.

257 Lauren E. Skelly et al., "High-Intensity Interval Exercise Induces 24-h Energy Expenditure Similar to Traditional Endurance Exercise Despite Reduced Time Commitment," Appl Physiol Nutr Metab 39, no 7 (2014): 845-848, doi: 10.1139/apnm-2013-0562.

258 "Hunter-Gatherer Culture," National Geographic, accessed April 6, 2023, https://www.nationalgeographic.org/encyclopedia/hunter-gatherer-culture/.

259 Iñigo San Millán, "Zone 2 Training for Endurance Athletes: Build Your Aerobic Capacity," Trainingpeaks online, accessed April 6, 2023, https://www.trainingpeaks.com/blog/zone-2-training-for-endurance-athletes/.

260 Peter Schnohr et al., "Various Leisure-Time Physical Activities Associated with Widely Divergent Life Expectancies: The Copenhagen City Heart Study," Mayo Clin Proc 98, no. 12 (2018): 1775-1785, doi: 10.1016/j.mayocp.2018.06.025.

261 "Sauna Health Benefits: Are Saunas Healthy or Harmful?" Harvard Health Publishing, Harvard Medical School online, last modified May 14, 2020, https://www.health.harvard.edu/staying-healthy/saunas-and-your-health.

262 Tanjaniina Laukkanen et al., "Sauna Bathing is Associated with Reduced Cardiovascular Mortality and Improves Risk Prediction in Men and Women: A Prospective Cohort Study," BMC Med 16, no. 1 (2018): 219, doi: 10.1186/s12916-018-1198-0.

263 James Roland, "8 Benefits of Sweating It Out with Hot Yoga," last modified September 11, 2019, https://www.healthline.com/health/hot-yoga-benefits.

264 Stacy D. Hunter et al., "Improvements in Glucose Tolerance with Bikram Yoga in Older Obese Adults: A Pilot Study," J Bodyw Mov Ther 17, no. 4 (2013): 404-407, doi: 10.1016/j.jbmt.2013.01.002.

265 Joanna Rymaszewska et al., "Efficacy of the Whole-Body Cryotherapy as Add-on Therapy to Pharmacological Treatment of Depression-A Randomized Controlled Trial," Front Psychiatry 11 (2020): 522, doi: 10.3389/fpsyt.2020.00522.

266 Ksenija Velickovic et al., "Low Temperature Exposure Induces Browning of Bone Marrow Stem Cell Derived Adipocytes in Vitro," Sci Rep 8, no. 1 (2018): 4974, doi: 10.1038/s41598-018-23267-9.

267 https://www.nih.gov/news-events/nih-research-matters/how-brown-fat-improves-metabolism.

268 Kristeen Cherney, "Cold Shower for Anxiety: Does It Help?" last modified June 22, 2020, https://www.healthline.com/health/anxiety/cold-shower-for-anxiety.

269 Sara Lindberg, "Ice Bath Benefits: What the Research Says," last modified April 9, 2020, https://www.healthline.com/health/exercise-fitness/ice-bath-benefits.

270 Matthias Wacker and Michael F. Holick, "Sunlight and Vitamin D: A Global Perspective for Health," Dermatoendocrinol 5, no. 1 (2013): 51-108, doi: 10.4161/derm.24494.

271 "Radiation: Ultraviolet (UV) radiation," World Health Organization online, March 9, 2016, https://www.who.int/news-room/questions-and-answers/item/radiation-ultraviolet-(uv); "Sunlight," Wikipedia, last modified March 15, 2023, https://en.wikipedia.org/wiki/Sunlight#cite_note-18.

272 Joseph Tafur and Paul J. Mills, "Low-Intensity Light Therapy: Exploring the Role of Redox Mechanisms," Photomed Laser Surg 26, no. 4 (2008): 323-328, doi: 10.1089/pho.2007.2184.

273 Johnjoe McFadded and Al-Khalili Jim, "The Origins of Quantum Biology," Proc Math Phys Eng Sci 474, no. 2220 (2018), doi: 10.1098/rspa.2018.0674.

274   Kim M. Pfotenhauer and Jay H. Shubrook, "Vitamin D Deficiency, Its Role in Health and Disease, and Current Supplementation Recommendations," Journal of Osteopathic Medicine 117, no. 5 (2017): 301, doi: 10.7556/jaoa.2017.055.

275   Miguel A. Maestro et al., "Vitamin D Receptor 2016: Novel Ligands and Structural Insights," Expert Opin Ther Pat 26, no. 11 (2016): 1291-1306, doi: 10.1080/13543776.2016.1216547.

276   "Vitamin D," National Health Institutes of Health, accessed April 6, 2023, https://ods.od.nih.gov/factsheets/VitaminD-HealthProfessional/; Shaima Sirjudeen, Iltaf Shah, and Asma Al Manhali, "A Narrative Role of Vitamin D and Its Receptor: With Current Evidence on the Gastric Tissues," Int J Mol Sci 20, no. 15 (2019): 3832, doi: 10.3390/ijms20153832.

277   Luna Vranić, Ivana Mikolašević, and Sandra Milić, "Vitamin D Deficiency: Consequence or Cause of Obesity?" Medicina (Kaunas) 55, no. 9 (2019): 541, doi: 10.3390/medicina55090541.

278   Mikael Häggström, "Establishment and Clinical Use of Reference Ranges," WikiJournal of Medicine 1, no. 1 (2014), doi: 10.15347/WJM/2014.003.

279   Martin Gaksch et al., "Vitamin D and Mortality: Individual Participant Data Meta-Analysis of Standardized 25-Hydroxyvitamin D in 26916 Individuals from a European Consortium," Meta-Analysis 12, no. 2 (2017): e017091, doi: 10.1371/journal.pone.0170791.

280   Maria-Antonia Serrano et al., "How Much Sun Is Good for Our Health?" last modified March 8, 2017, https://www.sciencedaily.com/releases/2017/03/170308083938.htm.

281   Andrei P. Sommer, "Mitochondrial Solar Sensitivity: Evolutionary and Biomedical Implications," Ann Transl Med 8, vol. 5 (2020): 161, doi: 10.21037/atm.2019.11.100.

282   Dmitriy Timerman et al., "Vitamin D Deficiency is Associated with a Worse Prognosis in Metastatic Melanoma," Oncotarget 8, no. 4 (2017): 6873-6882, doi: 10.18632/oncotarget.14316.

283   Dimitrios T. Papadimitriou, "The Big Vitamin D Mistake," J Prev Med Public Health 50, no. 4 (2017): 278-281, doi: 10.3961/jpmph.16.111.

284 Matthias Wacker and Michael F. Holick, "Sunlight and Vitamin D: A Global Perspective for Health," Dermatoendocrinol 5, no. 1 (2013): 51-108, doi: 10.4161/derm.24494.

285 Lars Alfredsson et al., "Insufficient Sun Exposure Has Become a Real Public Health Problem," Int J Environ Res Public Health 17, no. 14 (2020): 5014, doi: 10.3390/ijerph17145014.

286 Yoshihiro Sato et al., "Amelioration of Osteoporosis and Hypovitaminosis D by Sunlight Exposure in Stroke Patients," Neurology 61, no. 3 (2003): 338-342, doi: 10.1212/01.wnl.0000078892.24356.90.

287 Hannah Flynn, "What Do Studies Say About the Link Between Diabetes and Vitamin D Levels?" last modified January 21, 2022, https://www.medicalnewstoday.com/articles/what-do-studies-say-about-the-link-between-diabetes-and-vitamin-d-levels.

288 Mette Eskild Bornstedt et al., "Vitamin D Increases Glucose Stimulated Insulin Secretion from Insulin Producing Beta Cells (INS1E)," Int J Endocrinol Metab 17, no. 1 (2019): e74255, doi: 10.5812/ijem.74255.

289 Anastassios G. Pittas et al., "Vitamin D and Risk for Type 2 Diabetes in People with Prediabetes : A Systematic Review and Meta-analysis of Individual Participant Data From 3 Randomized Clinical Trials," Ann Intern Med 176, no. 3 (2023): 355-363, doi: 10.7326/M22-3018.

290 Johan Lundqvist, "Vitamin D as a Regulator of Steroidogenic Enzymes," last modified July 14, 2008, https://f1000research.com/articles/3-155/v1.

291 John E. Hall et al., "Obesity, Kidney Dysfunction and Hypertension: Mechanistic Links," Nat Rev Nephrol 15, no. 6 (2029): 367-385, doi: 10.1038/s41581-019-0145-4.

292 Thau L, Gandhi J, Sharma S. Physiology, Cortisol. [Updated 2022 Aug 29]. In: StatPearls [Internet]. Treasure Island (FL): StatPearls Publishing; 2023 Jan-. Available from: https://www.ncbi.nlm.nih.gov/books/NBK538239/.

293 B. Kloss et al., "The Drosophila Clock Gene Double-Time Encodes a Protein Closely Related to Human Casein Kinase Iepsilon," Cell 94, no. 1 (1998): 97-107, doi: 10.1016/s0092-8674(00)81225-8.

294 Ya Li et al., "Melatonin for the Prevention and Treatment of Cancer," Oncotarget 8, no. 24 (2017): 39896-39921, doi: 10.18632/oncotarget.16379.

295 Rüdiger Hardeland, "Neurobiology, Pathophysiology, and Treatment of Melatonin Deficiency and Dysfunction," ScientificWorldJournal (2012), doi: 10.1100/2012/640389; Iryna Rusanova et al., "Protective Effects of Melatonin on the Skin: Future Perspectives," Int J Mol Sci 20, no. 19 (2014): 4948, doi: 10.3390/ijms20194948.

296 Ewa Walecka-Kapica et al., "The Effect of Melatonin Supplementation on the Quality of Sleep and Weight Status in Postmenopausal Women," Prz Menopauzalny 13, no. 6 (2014): 334-338, doi: 10.5114/pm.2014.47986.

297 Kathryn L.G. Russart and Randy J. Nelson, "Light at Night as an Environmental Endocrine Disruptor," Physiol Behav 190 (2018): 82-89, doi: 10.1016/j.physbeh.2017.08.029.

298 "Blue Light Has a Dark Side," Harvard Health Publishing online, July 7, 2020, https://www.health.harvard.edu/staying-healthy/blue-light-has-a-dark-side.

299 Eloïse Sok-Paupardin, "The First European Standard for Daylight in Buildings," last modified December 12, 2018, https://www.sageglass.com/industry-insights/first-european-standard-daylight-buildings.

300 Gwen Dewar, "Why Kids Need Daylight to Thrive and Learn: The Benefits of Bright Light," last modified June 2019, https://parentingscience.com/kids-need-daylight/.

301 "Sleep Tips: 6 Steps to Better Sleep," Mayo Clinic online, May 7, 2022, https://www.mayoclinic.org/healthy-lifestyle/adult-health/in-depth/sleep/art-20048379.

302 Céline Tiffon, "The Impact of Nutrition and Environmental Epigenetics on Human Health and Disease," Int J Mol Sci 19, no. 11 (2018), 3425, doi: 10.3390/ijms19113425.

303 Agnese Mariotti, "The Effects of Chronic Stress on Health: New Insights into the Molecular Mechanisms of Brain–Body Communication," Future Sci OA 1 , no. 3 (2015): FSO23, doi: 10.4155/fso.15.21.

304 Bruce D. Perry, Child and Adolescent Psychopathology (New York: Wiley, 2017), 683-707.

305 Tarek Benameur, Maria A. Panaro, and Chiara Porro, "The Antiaging Role of Oxytocin," Neural Regen Res 16, no. 12 (2021): 2413-2414, doi: 10.4103/1673-5374.313030.

306. Dominique Turck et al. (eds), Nutrition and Growth: Yearbook 2002 (Basel, Switzerland, Karger Publishers, 2019), 94-113.
307. "Brain Architecture," Harvard University, accessed April 6, 2023, https://developingchild.harvard.edu/science/key-concepts/brain-architecture/.
308. Michelle Ward, "Early Love from Mothers Can Lead to Many Positives Later in Life for Kids," last modified May 10, 2020, https://www.ctvnews.ca/health/early-love-from-mothers-can-lead-to-many-positives-later-in-life-for-kids-1.4932851.
309. Bruce D. Perry, Child and Adolescent Psychopathology (Hoboken NJ, John Wiley & Sons), 93-129.
310. David Cantarero-Prieto, "Social Isolation and Multiple Chronic Diseases After Age 50: A European Macro-Regional Analysis," PLoS One 13, no. 10 (2018): e0205062, doi: 10.1371/journal.pone.0205062.
311. Edith Heard and Robert A. Martienssen, "Transgenerational Epigenetic Inheritance: Myths and Mechanisms," Cell 157, no. 1 (2014): 95-109, doi: 10.1016/j.cell.2014.02.045.
312. Vincent J. Felitti et al., "Relationship of Childhood Abuse and Household Dysfunction to Many of the Leading Causes of Death in Adults. The Adverse Childhood Experiences (ACE) Study, American Journal of Preventive Medicine 14, no. 4 (1998): 245-258, doi: 10.1016/S0749-3797(98)00017-8. PMID 9635069.
313. Donna Jackson Nakazawa, "7 Ways Childhood Adversity Changes a Child's Brain," last modfied September 8, 2016, https://acestoohigh.com/2016/09/08/7-ways-childhood-adversity-changes-a-childs-brain/.
314. Donna Jackson Nakazawa, "8 Ways People Recover from Post Childhood Adversity Syndrome," last modified September 18, 2016, https://acestoohigh.com/2016/09/18/8-ways-people-recover-from-post-childhood-adversity-syndrome/.
315. Michael Ungar, "Pathways to Resilience Among Children in Child Welfare, Corrections, Cental Health and Educational Settings: Navigation and Negotiation," Child & Youth Care Forum, 34, no. 6 (2005): 424-444, doi: 10.1007/s10566-005-7755-7.

316 Ann S. Masten and Jenifer L. Powell, Resilience and Vulnerability: Adaptation in the Context of Childhood Adversities (Cambridge University Press, 2003), 1-28..

317 Nicole K. Valtorta et al., "Loneliness and Social Isolation as Risk Factors for Coronary Heart Disease and Stroke: Systematic Review and Meta-Analysis of Longitudinal Observational Studies," Heart 102, no. 13 (2016): 1009-1116, doi: 10.1136/heartjnl-2015-308790.

318 Julianne Holt-Lunstad et al., "Loneliness and Social Isolation as Risk Factors for Mortality: A Meta-Analytic Review," Perspect Psychol Sci 10, no. 2 (2015): 227-237, doi: 10.1177/1745691614568352.

319 Mohd Razali Salleh, "Life Event, Stress and Illness," Malays J Med Sci 15, no. 4 (2008): 9-18, PMCID: PMC3341916, PMID: 22589633.

320 "Loneliness Is an International Issue," Campaign to End Loneliness online, October 2, 2013, https://www.campaigntoendloneliness.org/loneliness-international-issue/.

321 Clark Merrefield, "'Deaths of Despair': Research on Opioid Crisis Origins and the Link Between Minimum Wages and Suicide Reduction," last modified January 22, 2022, https://journalistsresource .org/economics/deaths-of-despair-opioid-minimum-wage-suicide/.

322 Daniel R. George et al., "Perceptions of Diseases of Despair by Members of Rural and Urban High-Prevalence Communities: A Qualitative Study," JAMA Netw Open 4, no. 7 (2021): e2118234, doi: 10.1001/jamanetworkopen.2021.18134.

323 "Suicide Statistics," American Foundation for Suicide Prevention," accessed April 6, 2023, https://afsp.org/suicide-statistics/.

324 Páraic S. O'Súilleabháin, Stephen A. Gallagher, and Andrew Steptoe, "Loneliness, Living Alone, and All-Cause Mortality: The Role of Emotional and Social Loneliness in the Elderly During 19 Years of Follow-Up," Psychosom Med 81, no. 6 (2019): 521-526, doi: 10.1097/PSY.0000000000000710.

325 "Chemistry of Love," ASDN, accessed April 6, 2023, https://asdn.net/asdn/chemistry/chemistry_of_love.php.

326 Julianne Holt-Lunstad, Timothy B. Smith, J. Bradley Layton, "Social Relationships and Mortality Risk: A Meta-Analytic Review," PLoS Med 7, no. 7 (2010): e1000316, doi: 10.1371/journal.pmed.1000316; Liz Mineo, "Good Genes are Nice, but Joy is Better," last modified April 11, 2017, https://news.harvard.edu/gazette/story/2017/04/over-nearly-80-years-harvard-study-has-been-showing-how-to-live-a-healthy-and-happy-life/.

327 Julianne Holt-Lunstad, Timothy B. Smith, J. Bradley Layton, "Social Relationships and Mortality Risk: A Meta-Analytic Review," PLoS Med 7, no. 7 (2010): e1000316, doi: 10.1371/journal.pmed.1000316.

328 Jens Brauer et al., "Frequency of Maternal Touch Predicts Resting Activity and Connectivity of the Developing Social Brain," Cerebral Cortex 26, no. 8 (2016): 3544-3552, doi: 10.1093/cercor/bhw137.

329 Suzanne Houk, "'Psychological Care of Infant and Child' A Reflection of its Author and his Times," accessed April 6, 2023, http://www.mathcs.duq.edu/~packer/DevPsych/Houk2000.html; Kathryn M. Bigelow and Edward K. Morris, "John B. Watson's Advice on Child Rearing: Some Historical Context," Behavioral Development Bulletin 10, no. 1 (2001): 26-30, doi: 10.1037/h0100479.

330 Evan L. Ardiel and Catherine H. Rankin, "The Importance of Touch in Development," Paediatrics & Child Health 15, no. 3 (2010): 153-156, doi: 10.1093/pch/15.3.153.

331 Alexander J. Horn and C. Sue Carter, "Love and Longevity: A Social Dependency Hypothesis," Comprehensive Psychoneuroendocrinology 8 (2021): 100088, doi: 10.1016/j.cpnec.2021.100088.

332 "How Does Physician Empathy Affect Patient Outcomes?" Gold Foundation online, July 3, 2013, https://www.gold-foundation.org/newsroom/blog/how-does-physician-empathy-affect-patient-outcomes/.

www.ingramcontent.com/pod-product-compliance
Lightning Source LLC
LaVergne TN
LVHW010203070526
838199LV00062B/4479